AF413027

Prognostic and Predictive Value of p53

EUROPEAN SCHOOL OF ONCOLOGY SCIENTIFIC UPDATES

Series Editors: U. Veronesi and M.S. Aapro

EUROPEAN SCHOOL OF ONCOLOGY SCIENTIFIC UPDATES, VOLUME 1

Prognostic and Predictive Value of p53

Edited by

Jan G.M. Klijn

Department of Medical Oncology
Rotterdam Cancer Institute (Daniel den Hoed Kliniek)
and University Hospital Rotterdam
Rotterdam, The Netherlands

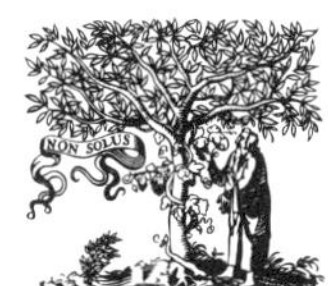

1997

AMSTERDAM - LAUSANNE - NEW YORK - OXFORD - SHANNON- SINGAPORE - TOKYO

ELSEVIER SCIENCE B.V.
Sara Burgerhartstraat 25
P.O. Box 211, 1000 AE Amsterdam, The Netherlands

ISBN: 0 444 82832 X

This book is printed on acid-free paper.

Printed in The Netherlands

The European School of Oncology gratefully acknowledges a joint sponsorship for the Task Force received from Pharmacia & Upjohn and Pharmacia Biotech.

Foreword

The European School of Oncology (ESO) is a non-governmental, non profit-making organisation, which was founded in 1982. It has since become a model for many other professional groups that need to provide timely information, education and training. The rate of progress in the diagnosis and treatment of cancer is so rapid that oncologists need continuous updating in order to provide their patients the best chances for palliation or cure. ESO recognises the multidisciplinary nature of cancer treatment, and its activities encompass all medical, nursing and technical specialities dealing with neoplastic diseases. Timeliness and scientific accuracy are the key factors behind the numerous activities of the School.

One of the many initiatives of ESO has been the institution of study groups, also called task forces, where leading experts exchange views on the state of the art of a given field, discuss controversies and new developments, and give opinions on future directions. These groups often publish a summary in a peer-reviewed journal, or excerpts of the discussions are presented as "Newsletters". The *Scientific Updates* are a series of books designed to disseminate the full results of such discussions. Each issue is under the responsibility of one or several volume editors, and contains the latest information on a particular topic.

To preserve the timeliness of the information, the ESO *Scientific Updates* utilise a simple layout and presentation to enable very rapid publication times, thus overcoming a common problem in the medical literature: that of the material being outdated even before publication.

The editors welcome suggestions for further issues and, together with the whole ESO staff, are ready to help interested parties in establishing new task force meetings. In this way the knowledge of new developments in all fields of oncology, from research through to nursing, can be shared. Education and training are important in helping reduce cancer-related mortality, and the ESO is firmly committed to achieving this aim.

Matti S. Aapro
ESO Scientific Updates
Series Editor

Umberto Veronesi
Chairman Scientific Committee
European School of Oncology

Contents

ESO Scientific Updates, Vol. 1
Prognostic and Predictive Value of p53
J.G.M. Klijn, editor

Introduction

Jan G.M. Klijn

Department of Medical Oncology, Rotterdam Cancer Institute (Daniel den Hoed Kliniek)
and University Hospital Rotterdam, The Netherlands

This first book volume of a new series of the European School of Oncology (ESO)
deals with one of the most important genes in the molecular genetics of human
cancer, namely p53. In about half of all cancers alterations of p53 or its pathway are observed. The cellular protein was first described in 1979, by a number
of investigators independently. Following the cloning of mouse p53 by Oren and
Levine in 1983, several laboratories initially demonstrated dominant oncogenic
activities of the gene. Later on, from 1989, p53 was recognised as a classic tumour suppressor gene based on the results of various studies by different research groups. Genetic alterations of p53 are mostly acquired during life and the
mutation spectrum differs between populations as a consequence of different local environmental carcinogenic factors. In a small minority of cancers the p53
gene defects are hereditary, resulting in the Li-Fraumeni syndrome.

Since the detection of the gene and its product various important functions
have been described. The gene appeared to be involved in cell cycle control,
DNA repair, apoptosis, cellular differentiation, senescence and angiogenesis.
The main function of normal p53 is to preserve genome integrity and the gene
has therefore been designated "guardian of the genome" by Lane et al. in 1992.
The year after p53 was proclaimed "gene of the year". During the last years
thousands of papers on p53 have appeared, underlining the importance of this
gene. Nevertheless, it is only in the last few years that we have learnt more
about the clinical aspects of p53 alterations due to the development of new
molecular genetic and immunological techniques that have greatly facilitated
clinical research.

In view of the rapidly increasing importance of p53 alterations for clinical
research and for the management of patients with cancer, the European School
of Oncology organised a Task Force Meeting in London on December 3-4, 1996.
During this interesting and lively meeting experts in different preclinical and
clinical disciplines and selected from various countries presented their data
followed by animated discussions. The following topics were discussed: 1) the
structure, different functions and interactions of p53; 2) relationship of p53 alterations with other tumour characteristics; 3) incidence and prognostic value of

p53 alterations with respect to a broad spectrum of tumour types and subgroups of patients; 4) predictive value of p53 with respect to response to endocrine therapy, chemotherapy and radiotherapy; 5) discrepancies in results of studies using different techniques for measuring p53 mutations and alterations of the p53 pathway; 6) p53 as a target for (potential) new treatment modalities. The main focus was on the predictive value of p53 regarding the response to different treatment modalities and its role in treatment resistance.

The final aim of the Task Force Meeting was the publication of an up-to-date review of this topic including contributions of the participating Task Force members, with references to the work of many others that were not present at the meeting. The papers were written in 1997 and resulted in the present publication. Covering a wide range of specialities, the contents of this book will be of interest to both preclinical and clinical researchers, as well as to students.

I would like to thank all contributors, the European School of Oncology, the sponsor, and, last but not least, Marije de Jager. Without her coordination and excellent editing and processing of the manuscripts the publication of this book would not have been possible.

ESO Scientific Updates, Vol. 1
Prognostic and Predictive Value of p53
J.G.M. Klijn, editor

The p53 Tumour Suppressor Gene: From Molecular Biology to Clinical Investigation

Thierry Soussi

Institut Curie, Paris, France

Introduction

Mammalian cells respond to DNA-damaging agents by activating cell cycle checkpoints. These control mechanisms determine temporary arrest at a specific stage of the cell cycle to allow the cell to correct possible defects [1]. At least two checkpoints monitor DNA damage: one at the G1/S transition and the other at the G2/M transition. The G1 checkpoint prevents replication of damaged DNA, whereas the G2/M transition is triggered by damaged and/or incompletely replicated DNA. Several findings have demonstrated that the product of the p53 tumour suppressor gene is responsible for the G1 checkpoint [2,3], and recent observations suggest that it may also play a role in regulating G2/M transition [4,5]. In response to genotoxic stress, the levels of p53 protein increase and this increase either determines a transient arrest of cell cycle progression in the G1 phase or triggers apoptosis.

The arrest in G1 is thought to give the cells time to repair critical damage before DNA replication occurs, thereby avoiding the propagation of genetic lesions to progeny cells. The cell cycle can resume once the damage has been repaired. This growth arrest is, at least in part, mediated by transcriptional activation of $p21^{WAF1/CIP1}$, which binds and inactivates the cyclin-dependent kinases required for cell progression [6]. Accordingly, homozygous deletion of p21 in mouse embryonic fibroblasts or in human colon cancer cells partially or completely abrogates radiation-induced G1 arrest mediated by p53 [7,8].

The mechanism by which p53 stimulates apoptosis is largely unknown. Several genes linked to apoptosis including bax [9] and Fas/APO-1 [10], are transactivated following p53 expression in some cell types, but whether the apoptotic properties of p53 are dependent on its sequence-specific transcriptional activation properties is controversial [11,12].

Address for correspondence: T. Soussi, UMR 218 du CNRS, Institut Curie, Pavillon Trouillet Rossignol, 26 rue d'Ulm, 75248 Paris cedex 05, France. Tel.: +33-1-42 34 65 11, Fax:+33-1-42 34 67 25, e-mail: thierry.soussi@curie.fr

The biochemical and genetic determinants that dictate which of the two pathways, death or arrest, will be chosen by a particular cell following p53 expression remain largely obscure.

In cells with no or mutated p53, DNA replication proceeds in the presence of a damaged template, thereby generating clones of genetically aberrant cells from which malignant clones may arise. Loss of the G1 checkpoint also results in genomic instability, as seen by the increase in the frequency of gene amplification in p53-defective cells [13,14]. Based on such findings, it has been proposed and is now largely accepted that the main function of normal p53 is to preserve genome integrity by acting as the "guardian of the genome" [15].

Further insights into the role of p53 have come from the study of null animals that lack endogenous p53 genes as a result of targeted gene disruption [16]. Mice homozygous for p53 null alleles have increased cancer predisposition, but are otherwise developmentally normal.

Association between p53 mutation and human cancer

Point mutations in the p53 gene have been found in most human cancers [17,18]. More than 10,000 different tumors have been analysed for p53 alteration and have led to the identification of mutations in many cancer types [19]. Their frequency varies from one type to another, but is in the order of 45-50% for all cancer types [19]. In general, these mutations are associated with a loss of the second allele of the gene. In certain specific types of cancer, p53 inactivation can be achieved through an epigenetic mechanism [20]. In cervical carcinoma, where the frequency of the p53 mutation is very low, p53 inactivation is considered to be due to the association of this cancer with human papillomavirus, which induces p53 protein degradation [21]. In soft tissue sarcoma, overexpression of the cellular protein mdm-2 leads to functional inactivation of p53 via the formation of a p53-mdm-2 inactive complex [22].

Another potential mutation-independent mechanism of p53 inactivation involves abnormal cytoplasmic sequestration of wild-type p53 with concomitant nuclear exclusion. This phenotype is present in 37% of inflammatory breast carcinomas and over 97% of undifferentiated neuroblastomas [23,24]. Recently it has been shown that this translocation compromises the suppressor function of p53, suggesting that it plays a role in the carcinogenesis of these tumours [25].

General interest of the study of p53 gene alterations

p53 mutation and patient prognosis

Is it possible to correlate p53 gene alterations with diagnostic or prognostic clinical parameters, and how may this information contribute to the treatment choice? Indeed, since Cattoreti's study in 1988 [26], the analysis of p53 overexpression in breast cancer shows that it occurs mainly in patients with a poor prognosis (absence of oestrogen receptors and high grade tumours). These findings in breast cancer have since been confirmed by molecular, immunohistochemical and serological approaches [27-35]. Thor et al. [36] reported that p53 gene alteration could be considered as a new, independent marker associated with poorer patient survival. A promising result was described by Allred et al. [28], who analysed a series of 700 breast cancer patients with no lymph node involvement (N0). Fifty-two percent (362/700) had a p53 alteration (measured mainly by immunohistochemistry). These patients had a much shorter relapse-free survival than those without p53 accumulation. If confirmed, this result could be very important because at present it is quite difficult to evaluate the prognosis of N0 breast cancer and the utility of adjuvant therapy following surgery. p53 analysis in these specific cases could be of major importance. Several studies indicate that there are some controversies concerning the immunohistochemical analysis of p53 alteration in breast cancer but a more recent study confirms that p53 could be an independent prognostic marker in lymph node-negative breast cancer patients [37].

Many similar studies have been conducted in other types of cancer but the results are not as clear-cut as in breast cancer, with the exception of colon [38] and bladder cancer [39,40]. Overall, tumours with p53 accumulation are generally high grade and more aggressive. For lung cancer, the results diverge as to whether p53 accumulation is related to poor patient prognosis [41,42]). As T. Mitsudomi [41] indicates, it is important to establish some level of standardisation so that studies of p53 accumulation will be comparable between series.

Heterogeneity of p53 mutant behaviour: clinical implications

p53 gene mutations are not random and are localised in the central region of the p53 protein. The importance of this region in p53 function has been suggested by several observations: i) the presence of 4 of the 5 evolutionarily conserved blocks [43]; ii) the high concentration of mutations in this region [17]; and iii) the fact that it is the binding site of SV40 T antigen [44,45]. The finding that p53 is never mutated in SV40-transformed cells suggests that its alteration occurs through interaction with AgT.

X-ray crystallography of p53 has been an important step in the understanding of the structure of this protein [46]. The central region (amino acids 102 to 292) has been crystallised in the form of a protein-DNA complex. This core region has been shown to include the following motifs: i) two antiparallel B sheets composed of 4 and 5 ß-strands, respectively. These two sheets form a kind of compact sandwich that holds the other elements; ii) a loop-sheet-helix motif (LSH) containing 3 ß-strands, an α-helix and the L1 loop; iii) an L2 loop containing a small helix; and iv) an L3 loop mainly composed of turns. It is quite remarkable to note the very good agreement between these various structural elements and the four evolutionarily conserved blocks (II to V). The LSH motif and the L3 helix are involved in direct DNA interaction (LSH with the major groove and L3 with the minor groove). The L2 loop is presumed to provide stabilisation by associating with the L3 loop. These two loops are held together by a zinc atom tetracoordinated to the following amino acids: Cys176 and His179 on the L2 loop and Cys278 and Cys242 on the L3 loop [46].

Analysis of the distribution of mutations in p53 shows a high concentration in the central region of the protein, and especially in the four blocks II-V which have been identified as the DNA binding region. In view of the 3-dimensional structure of the protein, it has been proposed that two classes of mutations can be predicted: class I mutations which affect the amino acids directly involved in the protein-DNA interaction (residues in the LSH and L3), and class II mutations which affect the amino acids involved in stabilisation of the 3-dimensional structure of the protein (residues in L2).

In fact, as described above, it has been established that mutant p53 can undergo conformational changes leading to its interaction with the heat shock protein hsp70, but also to altered accessibility to certain monoclonal antibodies such as PAb1620, which recognises a specific conformational epitope of wild-type p53, or PAb240, which recognises a cryptic epitope revealed in mutant p53 [47]. In reality the situation is not so simple, and there have been various reports of a certain degree of heterogeneity in the behaviour of different p53 mutants (see [48] for review). With the aim of analysing a possible correlation between conformational changes and loss in activity, Ory et al. [49] studied a library of 23 p53 proteins mutated in the 3 hot spot codons, Arg175, 248 and 273. The results show that these mutants may be classified into two different phenotypes, corresponding to the two classes discussed above. The phenotype PAb1620-/PAb240+/hsp70+ corresponds to all mutations found in codon 175 and to a single mutant in codon 273 (Arg → Pro), while phenotype PAb1620+/PAb240-/hsp70- corresponds to mutations in codons 248 and 273. No intermediate cases were found and each of these mutant p53 proteins had lost its transactivation and growth inhibition activities [49]. In fact, the conformational changes in p53 were dissected by a new battery of monoclonal antibodies directed against the central region of the protein [50]. All these antibodies recognise different epitopes in the central region of p53. Like PAb240, none of these antibodies was able to recognise native, wild-type p53. On the other hand, they were all able to recognise the category I mutants described above, suggesting that these mutants all undergo an overall conformational change that loosens the compact structure of the protein [50].

Moreover, analysis of the properties of the different mutant p53 proteins shows that not all mutations are equivalent [51-53]. Analysis of a series of p53 point mutants has revealed the potential for selection of the ability to transactivate some but not all cellular p53-response promoters. p53 mutant Pro175 and p53Leu181 are tumour-derived mutants which have retained the ability to activate expression of the cyclin-dependent kinase inhibitor p21$^{WAF1/CIP1}$, but Pro175 is defective in activation of the p53-responsive sequence derived from the bax promoter and the insulin-like growth factor binding protein 3 gene (IGF-BP3) promoter, while p53Leu181 shows loss of the ability to activate a promoter containing IGF-BP3 box B sequences [52]. These specific defects are correlated with the impaired apoptotic function displayed by these mutants, whereas they display a normal ability to induce G1 cell cycle arrest [52].

These observations are of key importance because they predict that tumours may behave differently according to the localisation of the mutation. In fact, recent studies have associated a poor prognosis for breast [33] or colon cancer [54] with specific p53 mutations.

p53 and hereditary cancers

Transgenic mice carrying a mutant p53 gene develop many types of cancer, with a high proportion of sarcomas [55]. This observation led various authors to study patients with Li-Fraumeni syndrome. This syndrome presents as a familial association of a broad spectrum of cancers including osteosarcomas, breast cancer, soft tissue sarcoma and leukaemias, appearing at a very early age. Statistical analysis predicts that 50% of these individuals will have a tumour before the age of 30, and 90% before the age of 70. Germ-line mutations in the p53 gene have been found in several families with this syndrome [56,57]. In all cases, there is a strict correlation between transmission of the mutant allele and development of a cancer.

Detection of germ-line mutations in the p53 gene in families at high risk of cancer should make it possible to follow the segregation of the mutation and to develop a new diagnostic approach to discover these mutations.

p53 mutations: a model for molecular epidemiology

Analysis of types of mutation in different types of tumour defines the mutational spectra according to the cancer under study. Generally speaking, there are two types of genetic alterations, those derived from endogenous processes resulting from errors occurring during the various biological processes linked to DNA metabolism, and those of exogenous origin involving environmental factors. The location and type of substitution occurring as a result of these two types of alterations are different. It is therefore possible to use the spectra of these mutations to study the aetiology of a cancer (see [58] for review).

Endogenous mutations

Analysis of all mutational events affecting the p53 gene shows that 42% are C → T transitions, 60% of which affect a CpG dinucleotide. It is well known that spontaneous deamination of 5-methylcytosine at these nucleotides may be an important cause of this type of transition. In fact, the three hot spot codons 175, 248 and 273 contain such a dinucleotide. More than 90% of the mutational events in these codons are compatible with a deamination phenomenon. This observation is confirmed by various studies showing that codons 248 and 273 are methylated *in vivo* [59,60]. Analysis of the mutational events in cancers such as colon cancer, malignant haemopathies or brain cancer (cancers known to be unrelated to exogenous carcinogens) shows that the mutation rate at the CpG dinucleotide is very high, thus suggesting that most of the mutations that alter the p53 gene in these cancers are due to endogenous processes related to the deamination of 5-methylcytosine.

Hepatocellular carcinoma and aflatoxin B1

In 1990 there were two reports of mutations in the p53 gene in hepatocarcinomas (HCC), with a predominance of the G → T transversion at the third base of codon 249 (Arg → Ser) [61,62]. In one report the patient series was from Mozambique, in the other from the Qidong province in China. These two regions are known for their consumption of food contaminated by the fungus *Aspergillus flavis*, producer of aflatoxin B1, which is a very potent hepatic carcinogen implicated in the development of HCC and known to interact synergistically with the hepatitis B virus. A worldwide epidemiological study has shown that the mutation in codon 249 is strictly specific to countries in which the food is contaminated by aflatoxin B1 [63]. In Mozambique, for example, more than 50% of the mutations were found in codon 249, while in Transkei, which borders on Mozambique (and which has a similar rate of chronic HBV infection), the mutation rate at codon 249 is less than 10%. In fact, in countries which do not consume contaminated food (including Europe and the USA), the rate of p53 mutations in HCC is low.

It has been demonstrated *in vitro* and *in vivo* that this phenomenon is due to a very high sensitivity of codon 249 to the action of aflatoxin B1 [64-66]. This observation, along with the fact that this mutation is quite deleterious to p53 function, explains the existence of this mutational hot spot [67].

Skin cancer and ultraviolet radiation

Brash et al. [68,69] have shown that in spinocellular skin cancer, C → T mutations predominate in pyrimidine dimers. It is well known that ultraviolet radiation, an aetiological agent of most skin cancers, acts directly on these dimers. A particular characteristic of the action of UV radiation is the change in the bases CC → TT, observed in Brash's series but also in other skin cancer series such as basocellular cancers [70]. In patients with genetic DNA repair deficiencies, such as xeroderma pigmentosum (XP), the phenotype is much more marked [71,72]. All mutations found in skin cancers are located on the pyrimidine dimers and 55% are tandem mutations CC → TT [73]. This type of mutation is very rarely found in internal cancers (less than 1%). In skin cancers from XP patients, more than 95% of the mutations are located on the noncoding strand of the p53 gene, while in other skin tumours and in internal cancers no special trends are observed. This result therefore suggests that there is preferential repair of the coding strand, which has been confirmed by Toranaletti and Pfeifer [74]. These authors showed that the repair rate of pyrimidine dimers in the p53 gene is highly variable, with a particularly low rate in the codons that are often mutated in skin cancer. Such p53 mutations seem to be very early events as they can be found both in precancerous lesions such as actinic keratosis [75] and in normal skin exposed to UV [76].

These results taken together (predominance of CC → TT lesions on the non-coding strand) were experimentally confirmed in animals carrying UV-induced tumours [77].

Bronchopulmonary cancers and smoking

The analysis of the mutational events that alter the p53 gene in lung cancer is a good example [78-82]. These mutations are frequently found in lung cancer and most are G → T transversions, with a minority of transition mutations (less than in other cancers). Moreover, most of the mutated guanines are on the noncoding strand of the gene. This observation is totally compatible with the role of exogenous carcinogens such as benzo(a)pyrene, present in cigarette smoke, and the observation that the noncoding strand is less efficiently repaired.

A recent study on bronchial cancers in radon miners revealed a mutational hot spot in codon 249 (16 of 29 mutations) [83]. The mutation differs from that seen in HCC because it affects the second base of codon 249 (AGG → ATG). This suggests that radon is responsible for this particular signature, since this mutation is found in less than 1% of other lung cancers. Nonetheless, this result should be interpreted with caution since some authors have suggested that this mutation is due to a mycotoxin synthesised by a fungus often found in the bronchi of radon miners [84].

p53 mutation in breast cancer

Breast cancer is the third most common tumour in the world and represents 9% of the global cancer burden. This percentage varies considerably around the world: in high-risk areas, such as North America and western Europe, breast cancer accounts for 1 in 3 female cancers, while in low-risk areas such as China and Japan, it accounts for only 1 in 8 to 1 in 16. The importance of environmental factors in the aetiology of breast cancer is demonstrated by the change in risk in migrant populations. Rates of breast cancer in European migrants to the USA evolve relatively rapidly toward those of the US population, but changes in migrant populations from China and Japan are less rapid.

Analyses of the pattern of p53 mutations in breast cancer have led to the discovery of substantial diversity of the mutational pattern among cohorts from various areas in the world (Table 1) [85]. This heterogeneity concerns i) the frequency of p53 mutations; ii) the frequency of frameshift mutations (deletions and insertions); and iii) the frequency of transversions.

The frequency of the p53 mutation could reflect the sensitivity of the various methods used in these studies. Nevertheless, different frequencies and patterns

Table 1. Mutations in the p53 gene in breast cancers from 16 populations: comparison with other cancers. The table is adapted from the review of Hartmann et al. [85], with permission. The data for other cancers are taken from the p53 database [125], except for data relating to Sweden which have been kindly provided by J. Bergh.

| Origin of patients | No. of mutations (%) | deletion or insertion (%) | Transition | | | Transversions | | | | ref |
			G:C->A:T at CpG	G:C->A:T non CpG	A:T->G:C	G:C->C:G	G:C->T:A	A:T->C:G	A:T->T:A	
All studies on breast cancer	29 %	17	24	18	13	7	10	5	5	
Aomori, Japan	15(56%)	26	20	20	7	13	7	7	0	[89]
Tokushima	26 (23%)	19	35	11	8	4	4	8	11	[90][126]
Sapporo	17 (71%)	0	41	17	18	6	0	12	6	[90]
Tokyo	29 (25%)	21	17	21	24	0	3	7	7	[127]
Kagoshima	13 (26%)	0	39	8	15	0	15	8	15	[128]
USA Midwest white	29 (30%)	38	21	21	3	7	0	3	7	[87, 129]
Detroit black	16 (34%)	6	31	13	32	6	6	6	0	[86]
New Orleans black/white	14 (15%)	14	14	57	15	0	0	0	0	[130]
San Francisco white	14 (24%)	7	14	7	28	28	21	0	0	[131]
San Diego white	31 (31%)	13	13	19	23	19	3	7	3	[132]
Tennessee white	18 (22%)	0	11	6	6	33	28	0	16	[133]
Scandinavia	50 (18%)	18	32	20	10	2	12	6	0	[27, 134]
Scotland	41 (30%)	7	15	17	10	10	22	14	5	[135]
France	30 (19%)	10	27	20	0	10	16	7	10	[136, 137]
Austria	14 (23%)	14	36	14	0	7	0	0	29	[88]
Sweden	88 (20%)	19	25	14	19	5	11	2	5	[33]
All p53 database	6278	9	26	18	11	8	16	4	6	[138]
Colon cancer	508	6	52	15	8	3	10	1	5	[138]
Lung cancer	652	12	12	14	8	12	34	3	5	[138]

were found among 6 populations analysed by the same laboratory using the same methodology, suggesting that other factors could be involved [86-90]. Blaszyk et al. reported some striking differences in mutation frequency within Japanese populations, but the reasons for such observations are unclear [90]. The unusually high frequency of deletions and insertions in rural Caucasian midwestern women compared to other populations is also difficult to explain, and could reflect exposure to particular environmental carcinogens [91]. A similar explanation can be advanced for the heterogeneous frequency of transitions and transversions (Table 1).

The pattern of p53 mutations in breast cancer is highly complex. The differences in these patterns of mutation in geographically and/or racially diverse populations reflect an intrinsic (endogenous) pattern of mutation plus exposure to particular environmental carcinogens.

p53 gene: a model for molecular epidemiology?

In order for a particular gene to be used in the study of the origin of mutagenesis in the human population, it must exhibit the following properties: i) it must be mutated in a large number of cancers; ii) the mutation rate must be high; iii) it must be altered mainly by point mutations; and iv) molecular analysis of the gene must be relatively easy to carry out (small size gene). At present, these characteristics are found in two genes, the Ha-ras oncogene and the p53 gene. One of the disadvantages of ras is the small number of codons (3) that are the target of mutations. In contrast, more than 100 of the 393 codons in the p53 gene can be modified. Moreover, the p53 gene is mutated in more than 50% of cancers. It is therefore possible to undertake molecular epidemiological studies with the aim of seeking specific signatures of certain carcinogens and demonstrating their role in the development of neoplasia [58].

p53 and response to therapy

p53 gene mutations may be associated with drug resistance in some tumours. Knowledge of the p53 mutations should therefore be taken into account in the therapeutic choice.

Lowe et al. [92] have reported a very interesting finding concerning p53. It has long been known that some antitumour agents such as fluorouracil and ionizing radiation act by inducing apoptosis in tumour cells. These investigators showed that cells expressing mutant p53 are totally resistant to apoptosis upon treatment, whereas cells expressing wild-type p53 are sensitive to these therapeutic agents. This finding was extended to other tumour cell types and to various DNA damaging agents [93-95]. This observation is of major interest as knowledge of the status of the p53 gene in a tumour allows to make a suitable treatment choice. Recently it has been shown that specific p53 mutations are associated with *de novo* resistance to doxorubicin in breast cancer patients [96].

p53 and therapy

The observations described above suggest that the reintroduction of wild-type p53 in tumour cells or the conversion of mutant p53 to a wild-type conformation could induce apoptosis in these cells. In fact, this hypothesis recently proved correct, as Fujiwara et al. [97] showed that infection of a cisplatin-resistant tumour with a recombinant adenovirus expressing wild-type p53 induced a return to chemosensitivity of the tumour, which was destroyed by apoptosis. This observation was extended to various types of cancer treated with either irradiation or chemotherapeutic agents [98,99]. Phase I retrovirus-mediated wild-type p53 gene therapy of lung cancer has recently been reported [100]. No clinically significant vector-related toxicity was noted. Local tumour regression was reported in 3 of 9 lung cancer patients who previously failed on conventional therapy.

Analysis of alterations in the p53 gene

Molecular analysis

PCR followed by sequence analysis enables direct study of the type of mutational event that altered the gene. In over 90% of cases, this event is a point mutation that alters a single nucleotide among the 23,000 in the gene. Unlike the ras gene, for which only 3 of the 189 codons are targets of oncogenic mutations, in the p53 gene mutations may occur in 90 of the 393 codons required for the synthesis of the protein. This high degree of heterogeneity makes diagnosis more difficult because the region to be analysed extends over almost the entire gene. Thus, molecular analysis of the p53 gene is somewhat tricky, and unsuited for routine diagnostic use. It is nonetheless essential for molecular epidemiological analyses in which it is important to determine the relationship between the type of cancer and the type of mutational event. Semi-direct detection methods such as SSCP (single strand conformation polymorphism), DGGE (denaturing gradient gel electrophoresis) and CDGE (constant denaturant gel electrophoresis) may enable selection of the region of the gene to be analysed. However, these methods are not 100% reliable (see [101] for comparison between SSCP and DGGE).

It is possible to imagine that in the not-so-distant future new technical advances in sequencing methods (such as sequencing by hybridisation on solid support) or in screening point mutations (such as ligase detection reaction) and associated techniques will permit routine molecular analysis.

Immunocytochemical approach

One of the significant properties of mutant p53 proteins is their extended half-life. In normal cells, p53 is undetectable because it has an extremely short half-life (15 to 20 min). In transformed cells, the mutant protein is much more stable, with a half-life of 4 to 12 hours, and it accumulates in the nucleus. It is therefore possible to perform an immunocytochemical analysis (coupled with a histological analysis) in tumour tissue to directly visualise this nuclear accumulation. Such an approach has been used in many different types of cancer with a generally good correlation between molecular analysis (presence of a mutation) and immunohistochemical analysis (overexpression of the mutant protein) [102,103]. The advantage of this approach is that it can be routinely used in histology laboratories. There are also a number of disadvantages, however, including the fact that mutations that abolish p53 expression (splicing signal mutations, nonsense mutations, insertions or deletions) do not produce the protein and therefore give a negative result. These types of mutations are found in 5% to 10% of cases. On the other hand, it is now known that tumours can overexpress p53 in the complete absence of mutations in any part of the gene. Since this overexpression is specific to tumour cells and does not affect normal tissue, this finding is generally considered to result from an alteration of p53 by unknown mechanisms. The problems in evaluating p53 overexpression in tumours have been addressed in several recent reviews [103].

In the past two years, new monoclonal antibodies against human p53 have been produced by several laboratories [104-108]. Their advantage is that they can be used for immunohistochemical diagnosis in highly varied conditions, such as detection of p53 in paraffin-embedded sections after fixation in formalin or Bouin's solution [108].

Serological analysis

Ten percent of breast cancer patients have anti-p53 antibodies in their serum [109]. This percentage reaches 20% in children with B lymphomas, while it is zero in patients with T lymphomas [110]. These studies, conducted during a lull in the scientific interest in p53, were reviewed more recently in the light of new knowledge on p53 inactivation and stabilisation. Anti-p53 antibodies have been found in most human cancers [31,111-114]. There is generally a good correlation between their frequency and that of p53 gene alterations [115]. In lung cancer, which has a high rate of p53 mutations, the frequency of these anti-p53 antibodies is high (24%) [116]. In prostate cancer, where the p53 mutation rate is low, or in mesotheliomas where it is nil, the incidence of seropositivity is very low. Several multifactorial studies show a very good correlation between the presence of anti-p53 antibodies, overexpression of the mutant protein in the tumour and the presence of a mutation in the gene [111,112,117]. In breast cancer, the prognostic value of p53-Ab was studied in 353 primary breast cancer patients. p53-Abs were detected in 42 cases (12%) and were negatively related to oestrogen and progesterone receptors [118]. The median duration of follow-up was 5.3 years. In actuarial analyses, the overall survival was worse in patients with p53-Ab ($p<10^{-4}$); in Cox's multivariate analysis, p53-Ab was an independent prognostic parameter [118].

Detailed analysis of these antibodies indicates that they recognise both wild-type and mutant p53 [31,116,117,119]. The epitopes are mainly located in the amino and carboxy terminal regions of the protein, regions that are not in the hot spot areas [31,116,117]. These immunodominant epitopes have also been detected in sera of mice hyperimmunised with wild-type p53 [107]. Taken together, these studies show that overexpression of the p53 protein in tumour cells is responsible for the appearance of auto-antibodies. Serological analysis has the following advantages: i) simplicity of analysis (ELISA); ii) no need for tumour tissue; iii) the possibility of following the fate of the antibodies during treatment of the patient. In addition, evaluation of p53-Ab could represent a very powerful tool for detecting infraclinical tumour lesions. Recently, p53-Abs were detected in sera of two patients who were heavy smokers without diagnosed lung malignancy [120]. Both these patients developed invasive squamous lung cancer 5 and 15 months after detection of serum p53-Ab. Since p53 alterations represent the most common, earliest genetic changes in lung carcinogenesis, it is suggested that p53-Ab detection represents a new and sensitive tool for detection of preneoplastic and microinvasive bronchial lesions in patients with a high risk of lung cancer, i.e., heavy smokers. This is supported by the recent observation that p53-Abs can be detected in sera of workers exposed to vinyl chloride and highly susceptible to developing angiosarcoma of the liver [121].

Functional assay

A functional assay for p53 mutations has been described [122]. Mutations are detected by assaying the transactivational activity of p53 protein in yeast. This test was used for detection of germ-line p53 mutations [123], but recent improvement in the test has led to its use in analysis of surgical specimens of tumour tissue [124].

Conclusions and perspectives

In addition to our knowledge of the p53 status of the patient and its clinical consequences, these studies provide considerable information and material concerning p53 function. It is clear that not all of these mutations are equivalent in terms of biological activity. It is now necessary to perform more basic research to elucidate such p53 mutant activity and its relationship with the transformed phenotype. All these efforts highlight one of the most exciting aspects of p53 studies, i.e., the constant exchange between basic research and clinical studies. It is expected that this knowledge will be of future benefit to the patient by enabling earlier, more precise diagnosis, and by generating new therapeutic approaches.

Acknowledgements

I am grateful to J. Bram for reading the manuscript. I also thank J. Bergh and S. Summer for their permission to use their data on p53 mutations. Research in the author's laboratory has been supported by grants from the Association de Recherche sur le Cancer, the Ligue Nationale contre le Cancer (Comité de Paris and Comité Nationale) and the MGEN.

References

1   Hartwell L, Weinert T, Kadyk L, Garvik B. Cell cycle checkpoints, genomic integrity, and cancer. Cold Spring Harb Symp Quant Bio 3 1994; 59: 259-63

2   Kastan MB, Onyekwere O, Sidransky D, Vogelstein B, Craig RW. Participation of p53 protein in the cellular response to DNA damage. Cancer Res 1991; 51: 6304-11

3   Kuerbitz SJ, Plunkett BS, Walsh WV, Kastan MB. Wild-type p53 is a cell cycle checkpoint determinant following irradiation. Proc Natl Acad Sci USA 1992; 89: 7491-5

4   Guillouf C, Rosselli F, Krishnaraju K, Moustacchi E, Hoffman B, Liebermann DA. p53 involvement in control of G2 exit of the cell cycle: role in DNA damage-induced apoptosis. Oncogene 1995; 10: 2263-70

5   Stewart N, Hicks GG, Paraskevas F, Mowat M. Evidence for a second cell cycle block at G2/M by p53. Oncogene 1995; 10: 109-15

6   El-Deiry WS, Tokino T, Velculescu VE et al. WAF1, a potential mediator of p53 tumor suppression. Cell 1993; 75: 817-25

7   Waldman T, Kinzler KW, Vogelstein B. p21 is necessary for the p53-mediated G(1) arrest in human cancer cells. Cancer Res 1995; 55: 5187-90

8   Deng CX, Zhang PM, Harper JW, Elledge SJ, Leder P. Mice lacking p21(CIP1/WAF1) undergo normal development, but are defective in G1 checkpoint control. Cell 1995; 82: 675-84

9   Miyashita T, Reed JC. Tumor suppressor p53 is a direct transcriptional activator of the human bax gene. Cell 1995; 80: 293-9

10   Owenschaub LB, Zhang W, Cusack JC et al. Wild-type human p53 and a temperature-sensitive mutant induce Fas/APO-1 expression. Mol Cell Biol 1995; 15: 3032-40

11   Haupt Y, Rowan S, Shaulian E, Vousden KH, Oren M. Induction of apoptosis in HeLa cells by trans-activation-deficient p53. Gene Develop 1995; 9: 2170-83

12   Sabbatini P, Lin JY, Levine AJ, White E. Essential role for p53-mediated transcription in E1A-induced apoptosis. Gene Develop 1995; 9: 2184-92

13   Livingstone LR, White A, Sprouse J, Livanos E, Jacks T, Tlsty TD. Altered cell cycle arrest and gene amplification potential accompany loss of wild-type p53. Cell 1992; 70: 923-35

14   Yin YX, Tainsky MA, Bischoff FZ, Strong LC, Wahl GM. Wild-type p53 restores cell cycle control and inhibits gene amplification in cells with mutant p53 alleles. Cell 1992; 70: 937-48

15   Lane D. p53, guardian of the genome. Nature 1992; 358: 15-6

16   Donehower LA, Harvey M, Slagle BL et al. Mice deficient for p53 are developmentally normal but susceptible to spontaneous tumours. Nature 1992; 356: 215-21

17   Caron de Fromentel C, Soussi T. TP53 Tumor suppressor gene: a model for investigating human mutagenesis. Genes Chrom Cancer 1992; 4: 1-15

18   Hollstein M, Sidransky D, Vogelstein B, Harris CC. p53 mutations in human cancers. Science 1991; 253: 49-53

19   Greenblatt MS, Bennett WP, Hollstein M, Harris CC. Mutations in the p53 tumor suppressor gene: clues to cancer etiology and molecular pathogenesis. Cancer Res 1994; 54: 4855-78

20   Soussi T. The p53 tumour supressor gene: from molecular biology to clinical investigation. In: Cowell JK, ed. Molecular genetics of cancer. Oxford: Bios Scientific Publishers Limited, 1995; 135-78

21   Crook T, Wrede D, Tidy JA, Mason WP, Evans DJ, Vousden KH. Clonal p53 mutation in primary cervical cancer - association with human-papillomavirus-negative tumours. Lancet 1992; 339: 1070-3

22   Cordon-Cardo C, Latres E, Drobnjak M et al. Molecular abnormalities of mdm2 and p53 genes in adult soft tissue sarcomas. Cancer Res 1994; 54: 794-9

23   Moll UM, Riou G, Levine AJ. Two distinct mechanisms alter p53 in breast cancer - mutation and nuclear exclusion. Proc Natl Acad Sci USA 1992; 89: 7262-6

24   Moll UM, Laquaglia M, Benard J, Riou G. Wild-type p53 protein undergoes cytoplasmic sequestration in undifferentiated neuroblastomas but not in differentiated tumors. Proc Natl Acad Sci USA. 1995; 92: 4407-11

25   Moll UM, Ostermeyer AG, Haladay R, Winkfield B, Frazier M, Zambetti G. Cytoplasmic sequestration of wild-type p53 protein impairs the G(1) checkpoint after DNA damage. Mol Cell Biol 1996; 16: 1126-37

26   Cattoretti G, Rilke F, Andrealo S, D'Amato L, Delia D. p53 expression in breast cancer. Int J Cancer 1988; 41: 178-83

27   Andersen TI, Holm R, Nesland JM, Heimdal KR, Ottestad L, Børresen AL. Prognostic significance of TP53 alterations in breast carcinoma. Br J Cancer 1993; 68: 540-8

28   Allred DC, Clark GM, Elledge R et al. Association of p53 protein expression with tumor cell proliferation rate and clinical outcome in node-negative breast cancer. J Natl Cancer Inst 1993; 85: 200-6

29   Thor AD, Yandell DW. Prognostic significance of p53 overexpression in node-negative breast carcinoma - preliminary studies support cautious optimism. J Natl Cancer Inst 1993; 85: 176-7

30   Callahan R. p53 mutations, another breast cancer prognostic factor. J Natl Cancer Inst 1992; 84: 826-7

31   Schlichtholz B, Legros Y, Gillet D et al. The immune response to p53 in breast cancer patients is directed against immunodominant epitopes unrelated to the mutational hot spot. Cancer Res 1992; 52: 6380-4

32   Barnes DM, Dublin EA, Fisher CJ, Levison DA, Millis RR. Immunohistochemical detection of p53 protein in mammary carcinoma: an important new independent indicator of prognosis? Hum Pathol 1993; 24: 469-76

33   Bergh J, Norberg T, Sjogren S, Lindgren A, Holmberg L. Complete sequencing of the p53 gene provides prognostic information in breast cancer patients, particularly in relation to adjuvant systemic therapy and radiotherapy. Nature Med 1995; 1: 1029-34

34   Jansson T, Inganas M, Sjogren S et al. p53 status predicts survival in breast cancer patients treated with or without postoperative radiotherapy: a novel hypothesis based on clinical findings. J Clin Oncol 1995; 13: 2745-51

35   Silvestrini R, Benini E, Daidone MG et al. p53 as an independent prognostic marker in lymph node-negative breast cancer patients. J Natl Cancer Inst 1993; 85: 965-70

36   Thor AD, Moore DH, Edgerton SM et al. Accumulation of p53 tumor suppressor gene protein - an independent marker of prognosis in breast cancers. J Natl Cancer Inst 1992; 84: 845-55

37   Silvestrini R, Daidone MG, Benini E et al. Validation of P53 accumulation as a predictor of distant metastasis at 10 years of follow-up in 1400 node-negative breast cancers. Clin Cancer Res 1996; 2: 2007-13

38   Hamelin R, Laurent-Puig P, Olschwang S et al. Association of p53 mutations with short survival in colorectal cancer. Gastroenterology 1994; 106: 42-8

39   Lacombe L, Dalbagni G, Zhang ZF et al. Overexpression of p53 protein in a high-risk population of patients with superficial bladder cancer before and after Bacillus Calmette-Guerin therapy: Correlation to clinical outcome. J Clin Oncol 1996; 14: 2646-52

40   Sarkis AS, Dalbagni G, Cordoncardo C et al. Nuclear overexpression of p53-protein in transitional cell bladder carcinoma - a marker for disease progression. J Natl Cancer Inst 1993; 85: 53-9

41   Mitsudomi T. P53 in non-small-cell lung cancer - response. J Natl Cancer Inst 1994; 86: 802-3

42   Passlick B, Izbicki JR, Riethmuller G, Pantel K. P53 in non-small-cell lung cancer. J Natl Cancer Inst 1994; 86: 801-2

43   Soussi T, Caron de Fromentel C, May P. Structural aspects of the p53 protein in relation to gene evolution. Oncogene 1990; 5: 945-52

44   Tan TH, Wallis J, Levine AJ. Identification of the protein p53 domain involved in formation of the simian virus 40 large T-antigen-p53 protein complex. J Virol 1986; 59: 574-83

45   Jenkins JR, Chumakov P, Addison C, Stürzbzecher HW, Wade-Evans A. Two distinct regions of the murine p53 primary amino acid sequence are implicated in stable complex formation with simian virus 40 T antigen. J Virol 1988; 62: 3902-6

46   Cho YJ, Gorina S, Jeffrey PD, Pavletich NP. Crystal structure of a p53 tumor suppressor DNA complex: understanding tumorigenic mutations. Science 1994; 265: 346-55

47   Milner J. A conformation hypothesis for the suppressor and promoter functions of p53 in cell growth control and in cancer. Proc R Soc Lond [Biol] 1991; 245: 139-45

48   Soussi T, May P. Structural aspects of the p53 protein in relation to gene evolution: a second look. J Mol Biol. 1996; 260: 623-37

49   Ory K, Legros Y, Auguin C, Soussi T. Analysis of the most representative tumour-derived p53 mutants reveals that changes in protein conformation are not correlated with loss of transactivation or inhibition of cell proliferation. EMBO J 1994; 13: 3496-504

50   Legros Y, Meyer A, Ory K, Soussi T. Mutations in p53 produce a common conformational effect that can be detected with a panel of monoclonal antibodies directed toward the central part of the p53 protein. Oncogene 1994; 9: 3689-94

51   Rowan S, Ludwig RL, Haupt Y et al. Specific loss of apoptotic but not cell-cycle arrest function in a human tumor derived p53 mutant. EMBO J 1996; 15: 827-38

52   Ludwig RL, Bates S, Vousden KH. Differential activation of target cellular promoters by p53 mutants with impaired apoptotic function. Mol Cell Biol 1996; 16: 4952-60

53   Friedlander P, Haupt Y, Prives C, Oren M. A mutant p53 that discriminates between p53-responsive genes cannot induce apoptosis. Mol Cell Biol 1996; 16: 4961-71

54   Goh HS, Yao J, Smith DR. p53 point mutation and survival in colorectal cancer patients. Cancer Res 1995; 55: 5217-21

55   Lavigueur A, Maltby V, Mock D, Rossant J, Pawson T, Bernstein A. High incidence of lung, bone, and lymphoid tumors in transgenic mice overexpressing mutant alleles of the p53 oncogene. Mol Cell Biol 1989; 9: 3982-91

56   Srivastava S, Zou ZQ, Pirollo K, Blattner W, Chang EH. Germ-line transmission of a mutated p53 gene in a cancer-prone family with Li-Fraumeni syndrome. Nature 1990; 348: 747-9

57   Malkin D, Li FP, Strong LC et al. Germ line p53 mutations in a familial syndrome of breast cancer, sarcomas, and other neoplasms. Science 1990; 250: 1233-8

58   Soussi T. The p53 tumour suppressor gene: a model for molecular epidemiology of human cancer. Mol Med Today 1996; 2: 32-7

59   Magewu AN, Jones PA. Ubiquitous and tenacious methylation of the CpG site in codon 248 of the p53 gene may explain its frequent appearance as a mutational hot spot in human cancer. Mol Cell Biol 1994; 14: 4225-32

18   T. Soussi

60   Rideout WM, Coetzee GA, Olumi AF, Jones PA. 5-Methylcytosine as an endogenous mutagen in the human LDL receptor and p53 gene. Science 1990; 249: 1288-90
61   Hsu IC, Metcalf RA, Sun T, Welsh JA, Wang NJ, Harris CC. Mutational hotspot in the p53 gene in human hepatocellular carcinomas. Nature 1991; 350: 427-8
62   Bressac B, Kew M, Wands J, Ozturk M. Selective G-mutation to T-mutation of p53 gene in hepatocellular carcinoma from Southern Africa. Nature 1991; 350: 429-31
63   Ozturk M and others. p53 mutation in hepatocellular carcinoma after aflatoxin exposure. Lancet 1991; 338: 1356-9
64   Aguilar F, Harris CC, Sun T, Hollstein M, Cerutti P. Geographic variation of p53 mutational profile in nonmalignant human liver. Science 1994; 264: 1317-9
65   Aguilar F, Hussain SP, Cerutti P. Aflatoxin-B(1) induces the transversion of G->T in codon 249 of the p53 tumor suppressor gene in human hepatocytes. Proc Natl Acad Sci USA 1993; 90: 8586-90
66   Puisieux A, Lim S, Groopman J, Ozturk M. Selective targeting of p53 gene mutational hotspots in human cancers by etiologically defined carcinogens. Cancer Res 1991; 51: 6185-9
67   Ponchel F, Puisieux A, Tabone E et al. Hepatocarcinoma-specific mutant p53-249Ser induces mitotic activity but has no effect on transforming growth factor beta 1-mediated apoptosis. Cancer Res 1994; 54: 2064-8
68   Ziegler A, Leffell DJ, Kunala S et al. Mutation hotspots due to sunlight in the p53 gene of nonmelanoma skin cancers. Proc Natl Acad Sci USA 1993; 90: 4216-20
69   Brash DE, Rudolph JA, Simon JA et al. A role for sunlight in skin cancer - UV-induced p53 mutations in squamous cell carcinoma. Proc Natl Acad Sci USA 1991; 88: 10124-8
70   Rady P, Scinicariello F, Wagner RF, Tyring SK. p53 Mutations in basal cell carcinomas. Cancer Res 1992; 52: 3804-6
71   Sato M, Nishigori C, Zghal M, Yagi T, Takebe H. Ultraviolet-specific mutations in p53 gene in skin tumors in xeroderma pigmentosum patients. Cancer Res 1993; 53: 2944-6
72   Dumaz N, Drougard C, Sarasin A, Dayagrosjean L. Specific UV-induced mutation spectrum in the p53 gene of skin tumors from DNA-repair-deficient xeroderma pigmentosum patients. Proc Natl Acad Sci USA 1993; 90: 10529-33
73   Dumaz N, Stary A, Soussi T, Dayagrosjean L, Sarasin A. Can we predict solar ultraviolet radiation as the causal event in human tumours by analysing the mutation spectra of the p53 gene? Mutat Res 1994; 307: 375-86
74   Tornaletti S, Pfeifer GP. Slow repair of pyrimidine dimers at p53 mutation hotspots in skin cancer. Science 1994; 263: 1436-8
75   Ziegler A, Jonason AS, Leffell DJ et al. Sunburn and p53 in the onset of skin cancer. Nature 1994; 372: 773-6
76   Jonason AS, Kunala S, Price GJ et al. Frequent clones of p53-mutated keratinocytes in normal human skin. Proc Natl Acad Sci USA 1996; 93: 14025-9
77   Kress S, Sutter C, Strickland PT, Mukhtar H, Schweizer J, Schwarz M. Carcinogen-specific mutational pattern in the p53 gene in ultraviolet-B radiation-induced squamous cell carcinomas of mouse skin. Cancer Res 1992; 52: 6400-3
78   Chiba I, Takahashi T, Nau MM et al. Mutations in the p53 gene are frequent in primary, resected non-small-cell lung cancer. Oncogene 1990; 5: 1603-10
79   Iggo R, Gatter K, Bartek J, Lane D, Harris AL. Increased expression of mutant forms of p53 oncogene in primary lung cancer. Lancet 1990; 335: 675-9
80   Takahashi T, Takahashi T, Suzuki H et al. The p53 gene is very frequently mutated in small-cell lung cancer with a distinct nucleotide substitution pattern. Oncogene 1991; 6: 1775-8
81   Mitsudomi T, Steinberg SM, Nau MM et al. p53 gene mutations in non-small-cell lung cancer cell lines and their correlation with the presence of ras mutations and clinical features. Oncogene 1992; 7: 171-80

82   D'Amico D, Carbone D, Mitsudomi T et al. High frequency of somatically acquired p53 mutations in small-cell lung cancer cell lines and tumors. Oncogene 1992; 7: 339-46

83   Taylor JA, Watson MA, Devereux TR, Michels RY, Saccomanno G, Anderson M. P53 mutation hotspot in radon-associated lung cancer. Lancet 1994; 343: 86-7

84   Venitt S, Biggs PJ. Radon, mycotoxins, p53, and uranium mining. Lancet 1994; 343: 795

85   Hartmann A, Blaszyk H, Kovach JS, Sommer SS. The molecular epidemiology of P53 gene mutations in human breast cancer. Trends Genet 1997; 13: 27-33

86   Blaszyk H, Vaughn CB, Hartmann A et al. Novel pattern of p53 gene mutations in an American black cohort with high mortality from breast cancer. Lancet 1994; 343: 1195-7

87   Saitoh S, Cunningham J, Devries EMG et al. p53 gene mutations in breast cancers in midwestern US women: null as well as missense-type mutations are associated with poor prognosis. Oncogene 1994; 9: 2869-75

88   Hartmann A, Rosanelli G, Blaszyk H et al. Novel pattern of p53 mutation in breast cancers from Austrian women. J Clin Invest 1995; 95: 686-9

89   Hartmann A, Blaszyk H, Saitoh S et al. High frequency of p53 gene mutations in primary breast cancers in Japanese women, a low-incidence population. Br J Cancer 1996; 73: 896-901

90   Blaszyk H, Hartmann A, Tamura Y et al. Molecular epidemiology of breast cancers in northern and southern Japan: The frequency, clustering, and patterns of p53 gene mutations differ among these two low-risk populations. Oncogene 1996; 13: 2159-66

91   Sommer SS, Cunningham J, McGovern RM et al. Pattern of p53 gene mutations in breast cancers of women of the midwestern United States. J Natl Cancer Inst 1992; 84: 246-52

92   Lowe SW, Ruley HE, Jacks T, Housman DE. p53-dependent apoptosis modulates the cytotoxicity of anticancer agents. Cell 1993; 74: 957-67

93   Xia F, Wang X, Wang YH et al. Altered p53 status correlates with differences in sensitivity to radiation-induced mutation and apoptosis in two closely related human lymphoblast lines. Cancer Res 1995; 55: 12-5

94   Eliopoulos AG, Kerr DJ, Herod J et al. The control of apoptosis and drug resistance in ovarian cancer: influence of p53 and bcl-2. Oncogene 1995; 11: 1217-28

95   Fan SJ, El-Deiry WS, Bae I et al. p53 gene mutations are associated with decreased sensitivity of human lymphoma cells to DNA damaging agents. Cancer Res 1994; 54: 5824-30

96   Aas T, Borresen AL, Geisler S et al. Specific p53 mutations are associated with *de novo* resistance to doxorubicin in breast cancer patients. Nature Med 1996; 2: 811-4

97   Fujiwara T, Grimm EA, Mukhopadhyay T, Zhang WW, Owenschaub LB, Roth JA. Induction of chemosensitivity in human lung cancer cells in vivo by adenovirus-mediated transfer of the wild-type p53 gene. Cancer Res 1994; 54: 2287-91

98   Spitz FR, Nguyen D, Skibber JM, Meyn RE, Cristiano RJ, Roth JA. Adenoviral-mediated wild-type p53 gene expression sensitizes colorectal cancer cells to ionizing radiation. Clin Cancer Res 1996; 2: 1665-71

99   Yang B, Eshleman JR, Berger NA, Markowitz SD. Wild-type p53 protein potentiates cytotoxicity of therapeutic agents in human colon cancer cells. Clin Cancer Res 1996; 2: 1649-57

100 Roth JA, Nguyen D, Lawrence DD et al. Retrovirus-mediated wild-type p53 gene transfer to tumors of patients with lung cancer. Nature Med 1996; 2: 985-91

101 Moyret C, Theillet C, Laurant-Puig P, Moles JP, Thomas G, Hamelin R. Relative efficiency of denaturing gradient gel electrophoresis and single strand conformation polymorphism in the detection of mutations in exons 5 to 8 of the p53 gene. Oncogene 1994; 9: 1739-43

102 Dowell SP, Wilson POG, Derias NW, Lane DP, Hall PA. Clinical utility of the immu-
     nocytochemical detection of p53 protein in cytological specimens. Cancer Res 1994;
     54: 2914-8
103 Hall PA, Lane DP. P53 in tumour pathology - can we trust immunohistochemistry -
     revisited. J Pathol 1994; 172: 1-4
104 Vojtesek B, Bartek J, Midgley CA, Lane DP. An immunochemical analysis of the human
     nuclear phosphoprotein-p53 - New monoclonal antibodies and epitope mapping using
     recombinant-p53. J Immunol Methods 1992; 151: 237-44
105 Midgley CA, Fisher CJ, Bartek J, Vojtesek B, Lane D, Barnes D. Analysis of p53
     expression in human tumors: an antibody raised against human p53 expressed in *E.
     coli*. J Cell Science 1992; 101: 183-9
106 Legros Y, Lacabanne V, D'Agay MF, Larsen CJ, Pla M, Soussi T. Production of human
     p53 specific monoclonal antibodies and their use in immunohistochemical studies of
     tumor cells. Bull du Cancer 1993; 80: 102-10
107 Legros Y, Lafon C, Soussi T. Linear antigenic sites defined by the B-cell response to
     human p53 are localized predominantly in the amino and carboxy-termini of the pro-
     tein. Oncogene 1994; 9: 2071-6
108 Tenaud C, Negoescu A, Labatmoleur F, Legros Y, Soussi T, Brambilla E. Methods in
     pathology - p53 immunolabeling in archival paraffin-embedded tissues: optimal proto-
     col based on microwave heating for eight antibodies on lung carcinomas. Modern
     Pathol 1994; 7: 853-9
109 Crawford LV, Pim DC, Bulbrook RD. Detection of antibodies against the cellular pro-
     tein p53 in sera from patients with breast cancer. Int J Cancer 1982; 30: 403-8
110 Caron de Fromentel C, May-Levin F, Mouriesse H, Lemerle J, Chandrasekaran K, May
     P. Presence of circulating antibodies against cellular protein p53 in a notable propor-
     tion of children with B-cell lymphoma. Int J Cancer 1987; 39: 185-9
111 Davidoff AM, Iglehart JD, Marks JR. Immune response to p53 is dependent upon p53/
     HSP70 complexes in breast cancers. Proc Natl Acad Sci USA 1992; 89: 3439-42
112 Winter SF, Minna JD, Johnson BE, Takahashi T, Gazdar AF, Carbone DP. Develop-
     ment of antibodies against p53 in lung cancer patients appears to be dependent on the
     type of p53 mutation. Cancer Res 1992; 52: 4168-74
113 Hassapoglidoi S, Diamandis EP. Antibodies to the p53 tumor suppressor gene product
     quantified in cancer patients serum with a time-resolved immunofluorometry tech-
     nique. Clin Biochem 1992; 25: 445-9
114 Angelopoulou K, Diamandis EP, Sutherland DJA, Kellen JA, Bunting PS. Prevalence of
     serum antibodies against the p53 tumor suppressor gene protein in various cancers.
     Int J Cancer 1994; 58: 480-7
115 Lubin R, Schlichtholz B, Teillaud JL et al. p53 antibodies in patients with various
     types of cancer: assay, identification and characterization. Clin Cancer Res 1995; 1:
     1463-9
116 Schlichtholz B, Tredaniel J, Lubin R, Zalcman G, Hirsch A, Soussi T. Analyses of p53
     antibodies in sera of patients with lung carcinoma define immunodominant regions in
     the p53 protein. Br J Cancer 1994; 69: 809-16
117 Lubin R, Schlichtholz B, Bengoufa D et al. Analysis of p53 antibodies in patients with
     various cancers define B-cell epitopes of human p53 - distribution on primary struc-
     ture and exposure on protein surface. Cancer Res 1993; 53: 5872-6
118 Peyrat JP, Bonneterre J, Lubin R, Vanlemmens L, Fournier J, Soussi T. Prognostic sig-
     nificance of circulating p53 antibodies in patients undergoing surgery for locoregio-
     nal breast cancer. Lancet 1995; 345: 621-2
119 Labrecque S, Naor N, Thomson D, Matlashewski G. Analysis of the anti-p53 anti-
     body response in cancer patients. Cancer Res 1993; 53: 3468-71
120 Lubin R, Zalcman G, Bouchet L et al. Serum p53 antibodies as early markers of lung
     cancer. Nature Med 1995; 1: 701-2

121 Trivers GE, Cawley HL, Debenedetti VMG et al. Anti-p53 antibodies in sera of workers occupationally exposed to vinyl chloride. J Natl Cancer Inst 1995; 87: 1400-7

122 Ishioka C, Freburg T, Yan Y et al. Screening patients for heterozygotous p53 mutations using a functional assay in yeast. Nature Genetics 1993; 5: 124-9

123 Flaman JM, Frebourg T, Moreau V et al. A simple p53 functional assay for screening cell lines, blood, and tumors. Proc Natl Acad Sci USA 1995; 92: 3963-7

124 Tada M, Iggo RD, Ishii N et al. Clonality and stability of the p53 gene in human astrocytic tumor cells: quantitative analysis of p53 gene mutations by yeast functional assay. Int J Cancer 1996; 67: 447-50

125 Beroud C, Soussi T. p53 and APC gene mutations: Software and databases. Nucleic Acids Res 1997; 25: 138

126 Sasa M, Kondo K, Komaki K, Uyama T, Morimoto T, Monden Y. Frequency of spontaneous p53 mutations (CPG site) in breast cancer in Japan. Breast Cancer Res Treat 1993; 27: 247-52

127 Tsuda H, Iwaya K, Fukutomi T, Hirohashi S. p53 mutations and c-erbB-2 amplification in intraductal and invasive breast carcinomas of high histologic grade. Jpn J Cancer Res 1993; 84: 394-401

128 Umekita Y, Kobayashi K, Saheki T, Yoshida H. Nuclear accumulation of p53 protein correlates with mutations in the p53 gene on archival paraffin-embedded tissues of human breast cancer. Jpn J Cancer Res 1994; 85: 825-30

129 Kovach JS, Hartmann A, Blaszyk H, Cunningham J, Schaid D, Sommer SS. Mutation detection by highly sensitive methods indicates that p53 gene mutations in breast cancer can have important prognostic value (vol 93, pg 1093, 1996) (correction). Proc Natl Acad Sci USA 1996; 93: 3715

130 Shiao YH, Chen VW, Scheer WD, Wu XC, Correa P. Racial disparity in the association of p53 gene alterations with breast cancer survival. Cancer Res 1995; 55: 1485-90

131 Deng G, Chen LC, Schott DR et al. Loss of heterozygosity and p53 gene mutations in breast cancer. Cancer Res 1994; 54: 499-505

132 Glebov OK, Mckenzie KE, White CA, Sukumar S. Frequent p53 gene mutations and novel alleles in familial breast cancer. Cancer Res 1994; 54: 3703-9

133 Caleffi M, Teague MW, Jensen RA, Vnencakjones CL, Dupont WD, Parl FF. P53 gene mutations and steroid receptor status in breast cancer - clinicopathologic correlations and prognostic assessment. Cancer 1994; 73: 2147-56

134 Thorlacius S, Børresen AL, Eyfjord JE. Somatic p53 mutations in human breast carcinomas in an Icelandic population - a prognostic factor. Cancer Res 1993; 53: 1637-41

135 Coles C, Condie A, Chetty U, Steel CM, Evans HJ, Prosser J. p53 mutations in breast cancer. Cancer Res 1992; 52: 5291-8

136 Faille A, Decremoux P, Extra JM et al. p53 mutations and overexpression in locally advanced breast cancers. Br J Cancer 1994; 69: 1145-50

137 Mazars R, Spinardi L, Bencheikh M, Simonylafontaine J, Jeanteur P, Theillet C. p53 mutations occur in aggressive breast cancer. Cancer Res 1992; 52: 3918-23

138 Hainaut P, Soussi T, Shomer B et al. Database of p53 gene somatic mutations in human tumors and cell lines: Updated compilation and future prospects. Nucleic Acids Res 1997; 25: 151-7

ESO Scientific Updates, Vol. 1
Prognostic and Predictive Value of p53
J.G.M. Klijn, editor
© 1997 Elsevier Science B.V. All rights reserved

Subgroups of p53 Mutations May Predict the Clinical Behaviour of Cancers in the Breast and Colon and Contribute to Therapy Response

Anne-Lise Børresen-Dale

Department of Genetics, Institute for Cancer Research, The Norwegian Radium Hospital, Oslo, Norway

Breast and colon cancers are the two most common malignancies in the Western world. Early diagnosis to detect tumours at an early stage will greatly reduce the morbidity and mortality of the disease. Screening programmes using mammography and sigmoid colonoscopy have been introduced in many countries, and the number of cases detected with only local disease is increasing. Even in these cases the clinical outcome is highly variable. In the last decade, research has focused on the identification of patients at high risk of relapse to prevent undertreatment of aggressive disease, as well as exposure of patients with indolent tumours to toxicity, discomfort, and possible long-term effects of unnecessary therapy. At present, treatment decisions are based on traditional clinical and histopathological parameters, but these are far from being highly sensitive or specific. New prognostic biological markers that can select patients for specific therapeutic regimes are highly necessary. Alterations of the tumour suppressor gene p53 may represent such a marker.

Mutations that alter or eliminate p53 protein function are the most common genetic alterations observed in human cancers, and appear to be an almost universal step in the carcinogenic process [1,2]. The p53 gene encodes a nuclear phosphoprotein with multifunctional transcription activity that orchestrates the cellular response following DNA damage. p53 is responsible for maintaining genomic stability by blocking cell replication until the damage is repaired, or initiating apoptosis if the damage is too extensive for repair. Moreover, p53 plays a direct role in DNA repair, angiogenesis, senescence and differentiation [reviewed in 3-5].

Address for correspondence: A.-L. Børresen-Dale, Department of Genetics, Institute for Cancer Research, The Norwegian Radium Hospital, Montebello, 0310 Oslo, Norway. Tel.: +47-22-935677, Fax: +47-22-934440, e-mail: alb@radium.uio.no

Since loss of p53 function seems to abrogate both DNA repair and apoptosis, leading to accumulation of mutations and gene amplification, it seems reasonable to expect tumours with altered p53 function to be particularly aggressive. However, the high frequency of mutations distributed over a large region of the gene has led to the speculation that different mutations have different biological and biochemical properties. It has been observed in *in vitro* studies that not all mutations are functionally equivalent [6-8]. Since p53-dependent apoptosis has been implicated in mediating the toxicity of radiotherapy and chemotherapy [9-12], different mutations may also have a different impact on mediating resistance to such therapy.

Screening for p53 alterations

Screening for p53 alterations both at the protein level and the gene level in different tumours to evaluate its possible role as a prognostic and therapeutic marker has been a major task for many laboratories over the past years. Most studies have used immunohistochemistry (IHC) to detect accumulation of the p53 protein, which in normal cells is found in minute quantities. Many of the mutant proteins have an extended half-life and are detected by IHC. However, the correlation between p53 accumulation and p53 mutations is far from perfect. IHC detects most missense mutations but misses nonsense and all types of frameshift mutations. In addition IHC will detect an elevated expression of wild-type p53. The detection of p53 accumulation by IHC therefore has a somewhat different biological meaning, but may be as important as detection of mutations at the gene level. To accurately estimate the influence of p53 gene mutations on prognosis and to evaluate whether different mutants behave differently, both in relation to prognosis and therapy response, it is important to detect almost all mutations, even if they are present in small amounts, and to determine the exact nature of the mutation. The ideal technique for mutation detection should be fast and inexpensive, and be able to screen long stretches of the gene with high sensitivity and specificity. The development of automated direct DNA sequencing using fluorescent labelling has reduced the workload involved in screening for mutations. Nevertheless, in most laboratories DNA sequencing is not yet sufficiently rapid and cheap to be used in routine diagnostics. Besides, direct DNA sequencing is not able to detect mutations present in low numbers in the tumour investigated. We have found constant denaturant gel electrophoresis (CDGE) to be a suitable and reliable fast screening technique for the detection of p53 mutations [13-15]. CDGE represents an improvement of the conventional parallel denaturing gradient gel electrophoresis (DGGE). It is easy to perform, more reliable and reproducible than DGGE, and has a higher sensitivity in mutation detection than single strand conformation polymorphism (SSCP). In contrast to direct sequencing of PCR products, CDGE detects mutations present in as little as 1% of the cell population analysed. The migration pattern of a given fragment is sequence specific. A migration database may be used to predict the sequence alteration in a sample without sequencing. We have used this technique to screen large cohorts of patient material, both fresh frozen and formalin-fixed paraffin-embedded tissues, for mutations in the p53 gene.

p53 mutations and breast cancer prognosis

Relatively few studies have been published on the prognostic significance of p53 mutations in breast cancer [16-27] compared to studies using IHC detection. Among the IHC studies, which comprise more than 10,000 patients, a significant association with prognosis has been found in only one third. Mutation analyses in relation to prognosis have been performed in approximately 3000 patients up to now (Table 1). In all these studies except one, a significant association between the presence of mutations and a shorter survival was found.

Table 1. Frequency and prognostic value of p53 gene mutations in human breast carcinomas

Number of patients	Region of the gene screen	Mutation frequency(%)	Relative risk	P value recurrence	Ref.
96	exons 2, 5-9	19	NA	NA	16
101	exons 4-9	32	NA	NA	17
148	exons 5-8	18	NA	NA	18
200[1]	exons 5-9	14	2.2	0.01	19
163	exons 5-8	21	2.2	0.001	20
109	exons 5, 7-8	17	NA	0.001	21
186	exons 5-8	16	NA	n.s.	22
90	all exons	30	4.7	0.015	23
298	all exons	22	NA	0.002	24
142	exon 5-8	34	2.4[2]	0.013	25
727	exon 5 and 6	8	2.3	0.0001	26
600	exon 5-8	20	NA	0.012[3]	27

1) Only patients without axillary node involvement
2) Mutations combined with luminometric immunoassay
3) Recurrence for mutations in the Zn binding domain vs. mutations outside this region
NA = not analysed; n.s. = not significant

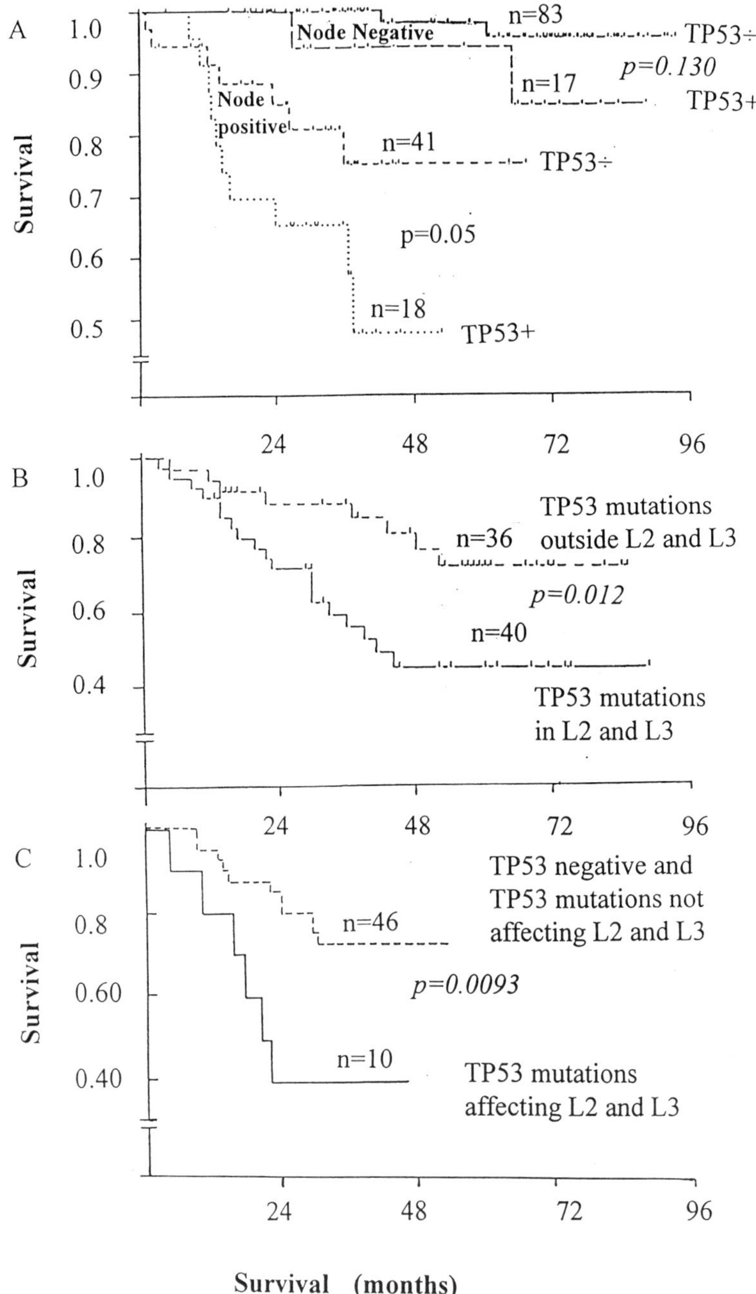

Fig. 1. Overall survival analyses (Kaplan-Meier plots) of breast cancer patients in relation to p53 status. The data shown are taken from A) Andersen et al. 1993 [20], B) Børresen et al. 1995 [27] and C) Aas et al. 1996 [40].

Differences in both frequency and survival rates have been observed between node-negative and node-positive patients with respect to p53 mutations. In our first study conducted in 1993 [20] a significant association with prognosis was seen only in the node-positive patients (Fig. 1A), although a trend towards a shorter survival was also observed in node-negative patients with a p53 mutation compared to those without. The number of cases in that study was, however, limited. In a much larger study of node-negative patients with a longer follow-up time [19] a significant association between p53 mutations and poor prognosis was found. In the study from Iceland [22], where patients with p53 mutations did not differ from patients without mutations with respect to survival, the mean follow-up time was 120 months compared to 32-72 months for all other studies. The treatment regimens for breast cancer have changed over time. The significant differences seen in survival between patients with p53-positive and negative tumours in the studies of more recently diagnosed patients, may reflect that the p53 status of the tumours alters the patients' response to therapy. The mechanism by which mutations in the p53 gene are associated with poorer patient survival is as yet unclear, although both growth advantages and resistance to therapy have been suggested.

Several *in vitro* and *in vivo* studies have shown that different mutations have different biological and biochemical effects, and the effect may also be cell-type dependent [6-8, 28-35]. The elucidation of the crystal structure of the protein [36,37] has provided a framework for understanding how these different mutations might inactivate its normal cellular function. The core domain of the protein, where most of the mutations reside, contains a scaffold made of a sandwich of antiparallel beta sheets supporting the DNA-binding surface. This surface comprises the two loops L2 and L3, which are held together by a zinc atom and interact with the major groove of the DNA, and a loop-sheet-helix motif which interacts with the minor groove. Furthermore, almost 50% of all mutations occur in the L2 or L3 domain. Tumours from 600 breast cancer patients from 6 different European countries have been analysed with respect to mutations in the p53 gene [20]. In this cohort of patients we found 119 with a p53 mutation in the tumour. The sequence alterations were determined in all of them. Deletions were found in 13 patients, all postmenopausal. When patients with missense mutations in whom survival data were available (76 cases) were stratified according to the different mutations found, recurrence of the disease was significantly more frequent among patients whose tumours had mutations in the L2 or L3 domain compared to those with mutations elsewhere (Fig. 1B). These domains correspond to residues 163-195 (parts of exon 5 and 6) and residues 236-251 (part of exon 7). Because the L2 and L3 loops contain residues involved in direct DNA contact as well as protein stabilisation, it is possible that these particular characteristics are responsible for the reduced survival rates. However, when we selected patients with mutations affecting residues involved in either DNA contact or protein stabilisation, they did not have a significantly decreased survival. This suggests that the observed effect on patient survival is specific for the L2 and L3 domain. The L2 and L3 loops have little regular secondary structure and rely extensively on various side chain and backbone interactions for structural activity. These interactions stabilise the zinc atom, hence anything that affects the L2/L3 interaction will affect this critical DNA contact. These results support the studies on cell lines concluding that different mutations are biologically different in terms of outcome. Since the measured endpoint in our study was disease relapse or death from the disease, we postulated that mutations in L2 and L3 were most likely indicative of failure to respond to therapy.

p53 mutations and response to therapy

Recent studies have shown mutations in the p53 gene or overexpression of the p53 protein not only to predict a poor prognosis, but also to predict the response to adjuvant radiotherapy or chemotherapy in breast cancer patients [24,38-40]. This is in agreement with several studies on p53-deficient mice and on human cell lines [10,41-43]. In a study of 63 patients with locally advanced breast cancer receiving doxorubicin monotherapy as first-line treatment we screened for mutations in the p53 gene [40]. Each patient underwent an open surgical biopsy before commencing on chemotherapy. Tumours were measured with regular intervals during treatment, and the clinical response was classified as partial response (PR), minimal change (MC), stable disease (SD) or progressive disease (PD). Of 18 patients (29%) that were found to have mutations in the p53 gene, four (22.2%) had PD during treatment compared with only two of 45 (4.4%) without mutations. In all four patients the mutation affected the zinc-binding domain (L3) of the p53 protein. In addition to these 63 patients, one patient with locally advanced disease receiving primary chemotherapy with 5-fluorouracil and mitomycin, had a mutation in the p53 gene affecting the L3 domain of the protein. She also had PD in response to chemotherapy. Thus mutations affecting the L3 loop were significantly associated with a risk of PD during treatment with doxorubicin (p<0.01). Survival analyses showed a significantly reduced survival rate for patients with mutations affecting the Zn-binding domains L2 and L3 compared to patients with mutations outside these regions or with no mutations at all (Fig. 1C). Our results support the hypothesis that functional p53 is of importance for the cytotoxic effect of this widely used drug.

Recently, studies on human fibroblast have shown that cell lines with defects in p53 function confer sensitisation to the anticancer agent paclitaxel (Taxol) that stabilises tubilin polymerisation [44]. Other studies using ovarian cancer cell lines defective in p53, or lymphoblastoid cells from Li-Fraumeni patients heterozygous for a p53 mutation, have failed to show such an enhanced sensitivity to the same drug [45,46].

In an ongoing study on ovarian cancer treated with paclitaxel and cisplatin in one treatment arm and cyclophosphamide (Sandozane) and cisplatin in the other, we have evaluated the effect of p53 mutations on patient response and survival. Preliminary findings show that in the cyclophosphamide group, 96%

of the patients with mutations in p53 had relapsed compared to 48% in the paclitaxel group. Patients without p53 mutations had a relapse rate of 60% in the cyclophosphamide group compared to 43% in the paclitaxel group [47]. These differences are statistically significant and indicate that patients with a mutated p53 gene have a much better effect of paclitaxel treatment than of cyclophosphamide treatment. In the group treated with cyclophosphamide, a trend towards a worse prognosis was seen in patients with a p53 mutation in the tumour compared to those without. No such difference was seen between patients with and without a p53 mutation in the paclitaxel-treated group.

p53 mutations and colon cancer prognosis

In human colorectal carcinomas mutations in the p53 gene occur late in tumour progression and are observed in 50-70% of the cases [5,6]. Some authors have observed that the presence of p53 mutations could be associated with poor prognosis in colorectal cancer [6-9] although others have failed to observe such an association [10,11], particularly when using immunohistochemistry to detect mutations [12-17]. To clarify the influence of different p53 mutations on long-term survival in patients with colorectal cancer, we performed mutation analyses using constant denaturant gel electrophoresis (CDGE) followed by sequencing in a series of 222 patients treated with surgery alone [48]. Mutations were found in 102 (46%) of the cases, more frequently in tumours located on the left side and in the rectum. Survival analyses indicated a shorter disease-free period and reduced overall survival for patients with mutations (Fig. 2A). When stratifying the mutations according to localisation, mutations affecting the L3 domain of the protein involved in zinc-binding gave a significantly shorter disease-free and overall survival (Fig. 2B). The patients in this study were treated with surgery alone. This indicates that mutations disrupting the L3 domain not only contribute to chemoresistance but also to a more aggressive tumour with growth advantages.

Conclusion

The results of the studies published so far strongly indicate that mutations in the p53 gene play a pivotal role in determining the biological behaviour of many different tumours including those of the breast and colon. Loss of normal p53 function seems to contribute to a more genetically unstable and aggressive phenotype. There are also several studies showing that loss of wild-type p53 function facilitates the development of neoplastic clones resistant to radiotherapy and to different chemotherapeutic agents. Certain mutations may be more important than others, but more studies are needed to verify these findings. Knowledge of a patient's p53 status, with respect to the presence of a mutation, to the specific nature of the lesion, and to the presence of a wild-type allele in addition to the mutated one, may accurately predict both the course of the disease and the response to different therapeutic interventions, especially those which induce apoptosis. In clinical trials evaluating new drugs and treatment strategies, the status of the p53 gene should be determined in order to evaluate whether in the future we will be able to select patients who will benefit most from a specific therapy.

Acknowledgements

Work referred to from the author's laboratory was supported by grants from The Norwegian Cancer Society. The author also wishes to thank all collaborators who contributed to papers 20, 21, 27, 40, 47, and 48.

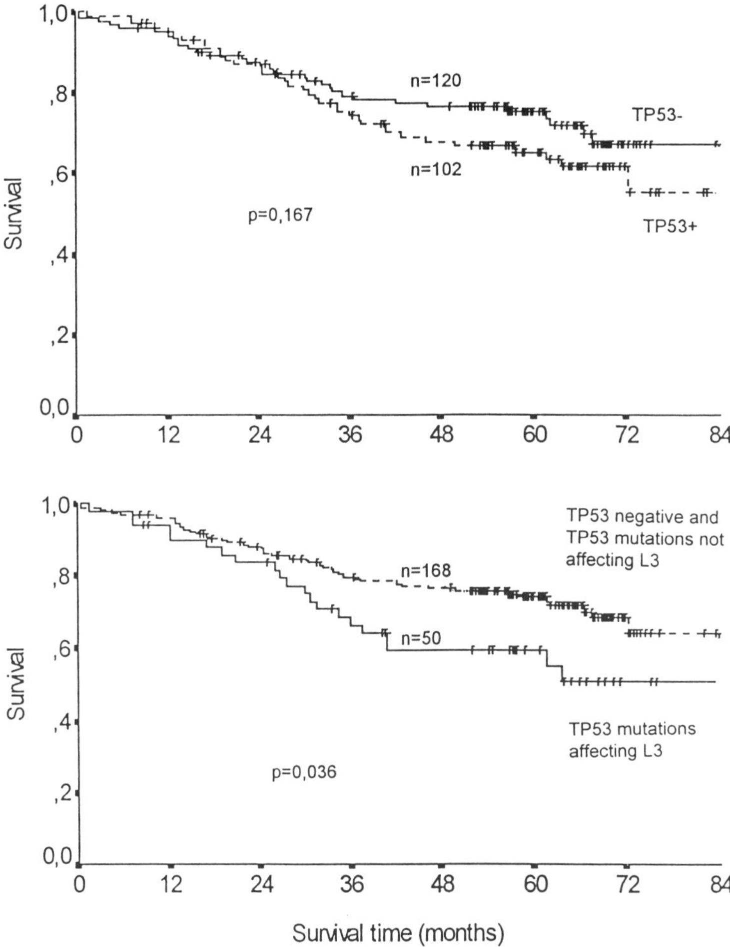

Fig. 2. Overall survival analyses (Kaplan-Meier plots) of colon cancer patients in relation to p53 status. The data are reproduced from Børresen et al. 1997 [48].

References

1   Donehower LA, Bradley A. The tumor suppressor p53. Biochim Biophys Acta 1993; 1155: 181-205
2   Harris CC, Hollstein M. Clinical implications of the p53 tumor suppressor gene. N Engl J Med 1993; 329: 1318-27
3   Ko LJ, Prives C. p53: puzzle and paradigm. Genes & Development 1996; 10: 1054-72
4   Kinzler KW, Vogelstein B. Life (and death) in malignant tumor. Nature 1996; 379: 19-20
5   Harris CC. Structure and function of the p53 tumor suppressor gene: Clues for rational cancer therapeutic strategies. J Natl Cancer Inst 1996; 88: 1442-55
6   Preudhomme C, Lepelley P, Vachee A et al. Relationship between p53 gene mutation and multidrug resistance (mdr1) gene expression in myelodysplastic syndromes. Leukemia 1993; 7: 1888-9
7   Pocard M, Chevillard S, Villaudy J, Poupon MF, Dutrillaux B, Remvikos Y. Different p53 mutations produce distinct effects on the ability of colon carcinoma cells to become blocked at the G1/S boundary after irradiation. Oncogene 1996; 12: 875-82
8   Iwamoto KS, Mizuno T, Ito T, Tsuyama N, Kyoizumi S, Seyama T. Gain-of-function p53 mutations enhance alteration of the T-cell receptor following X-irradiation, independently of the cell cycle and cell survival. Cancer Res 1996; 56: 3862-5
9   Kerr JFR, Winterford CM, Harmon BV. Apoptosis: its significance in cancer and cancer therapy. Cancer (Phila.) 1994; 73: 2013-26
10   Lowe SW, Ruley HE, Jacks T, Housman DE. p53-dependent apoptosis modulates the cytotoxicity of anticancer agents. Cell 1993; 74: 957-67
11   Kinzler KW, Vogelstein B. Cancer therapy meets p53. N Engl J Med 1994; 331: 49-50
12   Lowe S, Bodis S, McClatchy A et al. p53 status and the efficacy of cancer therapy *in vivo*. Science (Washington DC) 1994; 266: 807-10
13   Børresen A-L, Hovig E, Smith-Sørensen B et al. Constant denaturant gel electrophoresis as a rapid screening technique for p53 mutations. Proc Natl Acad Sci USA 1991; 88: 8405-9
14   Andersen TI, Børresen A-L. Alterations of the TP53 gene as a potential prognostic marker in breast carcinomas. Advantages of using constant denaturant gel electrophoresis in mutation detection. Diagn Mol Pathol 1995; 4(3): 203-11
15   Børresen A-L. Constant denaturant gel electrophoresis (CDGE) in mutation screening. In: Pfeifer GP, ed. Technologies for detection of DNA damage and mutations. New York: Plenum Press 1996; 267-79
16   Mazars R, Spinardi L, BenCheikh M, Simony-Lafontaine J, Jeanteur P, Theillet C. p53 mutations occur in aggressive breast cancer. Cancer Res 1992; 52: 3918-23
17   Tsuda H, Iwaya K, Fukutomi T, Hirohashi S. p53 mutations and c-erbB-2 amplification in intraductal and invasive breast carcinomas of high histologic grade. Jpn J Cancer Res 1993; 84: 394-401
18   Marchetti A, Buttitta F, Pellergrini S et al. p53 mutations and histological type of invasive breast carcinoma. Cancer Res 1993; 53: 4665-9
19   Elledge RM, Fuqua, SAW, Clark, GM, Pujol P, Allred DC, McGuire WL. Prognostic significance of p53 gene alterations in node-negative breast cancer. Breast Cancer Res Treatment 1993; 26: 225-35
20   Andersen TI, Holm R, Nesland JM, Heimdal KR, Ottestad L, Børresen A-L. Prognostic significance of TP53 alterations in breast carcinoma. Br J Cancer 1993; 68: 540-8
21   Thorlacius S, Børresen A-L, Eyfjörd, JE. Somatic p53 mutations in human breast carcinomas in an Icelandic population: A prognostic factor. Cancer Res 1993; 53: 1637-41
22   Gretarsdottir S, Tryggvadottir L, Jonasson JG et al.TP53 mutation analyses on breast carcinomas: a study of paraffin-embedded archival material. Br J Cancer 1996; 74: 555-61

23   Kovach JS, Hartmann A, Blaszyk H, Cunningham J, Schaid D, Sommer SS. Mutation detection by highly sensitive methods indicates that p53 mutations in breast cancer can have important prognostic value. Proc Natl Acad Sci USA 1996; 93: 1093-6
24   Bergh J, Norberg T, Sjögren S, Lindgren A, Holmberg L. Complete sequencing of the p53 gene provides prognostic information in breast cancer patients, particularly in relation to adjuvant systemic therapy and radiotherapy. Nature Medicine 1995; 1(10): 1029-34
25   DeWitte HH, Foekens JA, Lennerstrand J et al. Prognostic significance of TP53 accumulation in human primary breast cancer: comparison between a rapid quantitative immunoassay and SSCP analyses. Int J Cancer (Pred Oncol) 1996; 69: 125-30
26   Shadri R, Leong ASY, McCaul K, Firgaira FA, Setlur V, Horsfall DJ. Relationship between p53 gene abnormalities and other tumour characteristics in breast-cancer prognosis. Int J Cancer (Pred Oncol) 1996; 69: 135-41
27   Børresen A-L, Andersen TI, Cornelis RS. TP53 mutations and breast cancer prognosis: Particularly poor survival rates for cases with mutations in the zinc-binding domains. Genes Chromosome Cancer 1995; 14: 71-5
28   Hann BC, Lane DP. The dominating effect of mutant p53. Nat Genet 1995; 9: 221-2
29   Forrester K, Lupold SE, Ott VL et al. Effects of p53 mutants on wild-type p53-mediated transactivation are cell type dependent. Oncogene 1995; 10: 2103-11
30   Hsiao M, Low J, Dorn E et al. Gain-of-function mutations of the p53 gene induce lymphohematopoietic metastatic potential and tissue invasiveness. Am J Pathol 1994; 145: 702-14
31   Ossovskaya VS, Mazo IA, Chernov MV et al. Use of genetic suppressor elements to dissect distinct biological effects of separate p53 domains. Proc Natl Acad Sci USA 1996; 3: 10309-14
32   Kawamura M, Yamashita T, Segawa K, Kaneuchi M, Shindoh M, Fujinaga K. The 273rd codon mutants of p53 show growth modulation activities not correlated with p53-specific transactivation activity. Oncogene 1996; 12: 2361-7
33   Roemer K, Mueller-Lantzsch N. p53 transactivation domain mutant Q22, S23 is impaired for repression of promoters and mediation of apoptosis. Oncogene 1996; 12: 2069-79
34   Halevy O, Michalovitz D, Oren M. Different tumor-derived p53 mutants exhibit distinct biological activities. Science 1990; 250: 113-6
35   Kieser A, Weich HA, Brandner G, Marmè D, Kolch W. Mutant p53 potentiates protein kinase C induction of vascular endothelial growth factor expression. Oncogene 1994; 9: 963-9
36   Cho Y, Gorina S, Jeffrey PD, Pavletich NP. Crystal structure of a p53 tumor suppressor-DNA complex: Understanding tumorigenic mutations. Science 1994; 265: 346-55
37   Kussie PH, Gorina S, Marechal V et al. Structure of the MDM2 oncoprotein bound to the TP53 tumor suppressor transactivating domain. Science 1996; 274: 948-53
38   Jansson T, Inganäs M, Sjögren S et al. p53 status predicts survival in breast cancer patients treated with/without postoperative radiotherapy: A novel hypothesis based on clinical findings. J Clin Oncol 1995; 13: 2745-51
39   Stål O, Stenmark-Askmalm M, Wingren S et al. p53 expression and the result of adjuvant therapy of breast cancer. Acta Oncol 1995; 34: 767-70
40   Aas T, Børresen A-L, Geisler S et al. Specific p53 mutations are associated with de novo resistance to doxorubicin in breast cancer patients. Nature Medicine 1996; 2(7): 811-4
41   Lowe SW, Bodis S, McClatchey A et al. p53 status and the efficacy of cancer therapy in vivo. Science 1994; 266: 807-10
42   Hawkins DS, Demers GW, Galloway DA. Inactivation of p53 enhances sensitivity to multiple chemotherapeutic agents. Cancer Res 1996; 56: 892-8
43   Gudas JM, Nguyen H, Li T et al. Drug-resistant breast cancer cells frequently retain expression of a functional wild-type p53 protein. Carcinogenesis 1996; 17(7): 1417-27

44 Wahl AF, Donaldson KL, Fairchild C et al. Loss of normal p53 function confers sensitization to Taxol by increasing G2/M arrest and apoptosis. Nature Medicine 1996; 2(1): 72-9

45 Wu GS, El-Deiry WS. p53 and chemosensitivity. Nature Medicine 1996; 2(3): 255-6

46 Delia D, Mizutani S, Lamorte G, Goi K, Iwata S, Pierotti MA. p53 activity and chemotherapy. Nature Medicine 1996; 2(7): 724-5

47 Smith-Sørensen B, Kaern J, Holm R, Dørum A. Tropé C, Børresen-Dale A-L. Therapy effect of either paclitaxel or cyclophosphamide combination treatment in patients with epithelial ovarian cancer and relation to TP53 status. (in preparation)

48 Børresen-Dale A-L, Lothe RA, Meling GI, Hainault P, Torleiv OR, Skovlund E. TP53 and long term prognosis in colorectal cancer; mutations in the L3 Zn-binding domain predict poor survival. Clin Cancer Res 1997 (submitted)

ESO Scientific Updates, Vol. 1
Prognostic and Predictive Value of p53
J.G.M. Klijn, editor
© 1997 Elsevier Science B.V. All rights reserved

Determination and Use of p53 in the Management of Cancer Patients with Special Focus on Breast Cancer - A Review

Jonas Bergh

Department of Oncology, University Hospital of Uppsala, Uppsala, Sweden

General scientific background and economic reality

The basic sciences, with special reference to molecular biology, have progressed exponentially over the last two decades. This progress includes the discovery of oncogenes and tumour suppressor genes in human cancers. On the whole these findings have not been integrated into clinical medicine so far, with excellent areas of exception. The reasons for this lag phase are at least two-fold; i) scientific proof is still mainly lacking that diagnosis and therapy will be altered using these new tools, thus changing the clinical outcome for individual patients, and ii) physicians in clinical medicine need strong and repeated evidence that any new diagnostic and/or treatment modality is superior to current routines. A suitable example of delay in decision-making and different interpretation of scientific data could be the use of adjuvant polychemotherapy for premenopausal and node-positive patients resulting in a significant reduction in mortality, which was first described in 1977 [1]. A number of studies were initiated to repeat the data, which they did, but it was not until after the second overview that this type of therapy became generally accepted in some areas of the Scandinavian countries and the United Kingdom [2]. Apart from the above-mentioned points the strain on many economies in western Europe has, of course, added to the problems. In this atmosphere of general circumspection among physicians along with a restrained economic reality the scientific data must be very sound and must be proven to be significantly better that the currently used methods.

These background data ought to be known prior to any discussion of prognostic and predictive factors including p53, with special focus on human breast cancer.

Address for correspondence: J. Bergh, Department of Oncology, University of Uppsala, Akademiska sjukhuset, 751 85 Uppsala, Sweden.
Tel.: +46-18-66 54 92, Fax: +46-18-66 55 28, e-mail: Jonas.Bergh@Oncology.uu.se

General background of human breast cancer

Early diagnosis with mammography and adjuvant therapy, respectively, of patients with breast carcinoma have been seen to improve the relative survival by 25% [2,3]. At the first diagnosis of breast carcinoma the clinical scenario ranges from patients with small and indolent tumours who will be cured by a minor surgical intervention - some elderly women may not even require any surgery. For these patients the situation resembles that of prostatic carcinoma, that is, certain tumours seem to lack a truly malignant potential [4]. At the other end of the primary breast carcinoma spectrum are patients with rapidly progressing inflammatory breast carcinomas or patients with malignant tumours with more than 10 positive axillary lymph nodes at the time of diagnosis. When standard therapy is used the 5-year survival will be in the order of 5% to 10% for the inflammatory breast carcinomas, and 30% to 40% for the latter group. In many countries today these high-risk groups of patients are offered inclusion in clinical trials utilising different high-dose regimens with or without autologous bone marrow support strategies.

Prognostic and predictive factors

In view of the markedly dissimilar risks, the classification of breast cancer patients should be highly accurate. To make the issue even more complex, however, the bulk of patients are in between these extremes. There are a number of prognostic markers identifying groups of patients with different risk profiles (Table 1). Yet at present none of the currently used markers have the capacity to outline the individual risk profile with very high sensitivity and specificity.

Table 1. Prognostic factors needed for standard care

TNM stage
Histological grading system
Sex steroid receptors (oestrogen and progesterone)
Ploidy
S-phase

Investigational prognostic factors

Oncogene products (c-erbB2, int2, c-myc)
Tumour suppressor genes (p53, Rb).
Angiogenesis
NM23
Proteolytic enzymes (Cathepsin-D, urokinase)

One may rightly wonder whether there is a need for new prognostic markers before we have learnt how to optimally use the currently available ones. A not uncommon view is that the latter should thoroughly be tested in prospective and controlled studies to determine their value before introducing any new markers.

Factors delineating a prognosis with respect to the response to different therapeutic modalities used in oncology are designated "predictive factors". Examples of predictive factors are oestrogen and progesterone receptor status [5], e.g. an oestrogen and progesterone receptor-positive breast carcinoma has a 50% to 70% chance to respond to hormonal therapy whereas this response would be only 5% to 10% in hormone receptor-negative tumours. Increased expression of c-erbB-2, homologous to the epidermal growth factor receptor, has been claimed to be associated with a limited effect of adjuvant therapy with cyclophosphamide, methotrexate and 5-fluorouracil [6,7], while other studies have yielded partially opposite findings [8-10]. Furthermore, c-erbB-2 overexpression has recently been described as being associated with a decreased benefit from adjuvant tamoxifen for node-negative patients [11]. p53 has also been described as a potential predictive factor, but the number of clinical studies covering this issue are still limited. The basic characteristics of p53, its prognostic value and possible predictive value will be discussed in the following sections.

Basic information on p53

A huge interest has been and is still focused on the tumour suppressor gene p53, which was initially described as an oncogene. In 1995 about 150 scientific reports were published monthly on p53 [12]. The central function of the p53 gene is underlined by the fact that in 1992 it was designated as "guardian of the genome" [13]. p53 is involved cell cycle control, apoptosis, gene transcription, chromosomal segregation and genomic stability [14].

The p53 gene is located on the short arm of chromosome 17, band 13.1 [15,16]. The protein encoded by the gene consists of 393 amino acids. The p53 gene consists of 5 evolutionarily conserved regions [17]. The tertiary structure is largely known and the exact binding positions of several proteins including murine double minute-2 (mdm-2) to p53 have been disclosed [18-20]. The DNA binding region is located between amino acids 102 and 292. p53 can be inactivated by somatic or germ-line mutations (deletions of one or both alleles, nonsense, missense and splice mutations), by binding to certain viral oncoproteins (human papillomavirus protein E6, simian virus-40 large T antigen, hepatitis B viral X protein, adenovirus protein E1A) and to the protein from the oncogene mdm-2 [14,21] (Fig. 1). Patients with germ-line p53 mutations (Li-Fraumeni syndrome) have an increased risk of developing breast carcinoma, soft tissue sarcoma, adrenocortical carcinoma, gastrointestinal tract carcinomas, lung carcinoma and melanoma [26,27]. Mice with induced deficiency of both alleles of

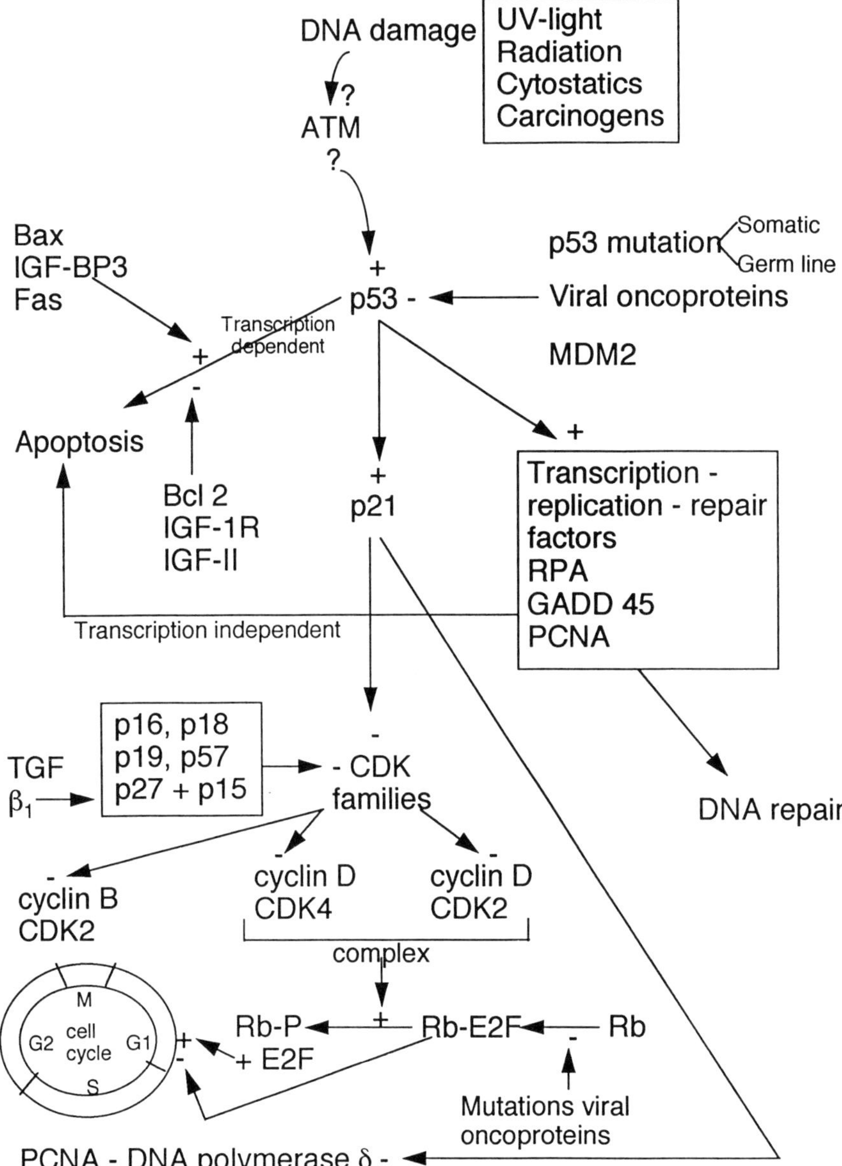

Fig. 1. Schematic illustration of the activation of p53 and its downstream mediators. ATM: ataxia telangiectasia gene product; CDK: cyclin-dependent kinase; E2F: transcription factor; GADD45: growth arrest and DNA damage factor; IGF-BP3: insulin-like growth factor binding protein 3; PCNA: proliferating cell nuclear antigen; Rb: retinoblastoma tumour suppressor; RPA: replicating protein antigen; TGF: transforming growth factor. Modified from Chang et al. [22], Stinchcomb [23], Harris [14], Norberg et al. [24], Velculescu & El-Deiry [25].

p53 develop lymphomas and sarcomas and in one study all animals were described to be dead within 2 years. Seventy-five percent developed tumours before the age of 6 months [28].

UV-light, radiation, carcinogens and cytostatic drugs can activate p53 and double strand breaks have been demonstrated to enhance p53 protein levels (Fig. 1) [14]. The p53 levels are elevated due to increased mRNA translation and extension of the half-life of the protein [12]. The activation of p53 may be preceded by or may involve the ataxia-telangiectasia (AT) protein. The potential link between p53 and AT is interesting because patients with AT have a markedly increased sensitivity to radiation, most likely due to deficient checkpoint controls in G1, S-phase and G2 after radiation [29-31].

Induction of p53 leads to activation and transcription of a number of factors including growth arrest and DNA damage factor (GADD45), mdm-2, bax and p21. The increased levels of the p53 protein can result in apoptosis, cell cycle arrest or DNA repair. The mechanisms for pathway selection are not known. p21 binds and inhibits cyclin-dependent kinases (cdk), which will prevent the transition from G1 to S-phase in the cell cycle. To make it even more complex, the cdks are inhibited by p16, p18, p19, p57, p27 + p15, and p21 (Fig. 1). The apoptotic pathway involves the balance between bax, insulin-like growth factor binding protein 3 (IGF-BP3) and fas, which promote apoptosis, versus bcl-2, IGF-1R and IGF II, which may block this pathway. Furthermore, bax has recently been demonstrated to act as a tumour suppressor [32].

Methods for p53 determination: immunohistochemistry and molecular biology

A number of techniques have been used to identify p53 alterations in tumours, in particular genetic analyses or immunohistochemistry for the demonstration of the p53 protein. Sequencing is relatively complex, time-consuming and expensive. Immunohistochemistry on the other hand is more commonly used because it is a rapid, inexpensive and convenient method for p53 detection. However, immunohistochemistry may have some potential shortcomings that will be discussed in the following paragraphs.

Most of the commonly used antibodies for immunohistochemical p53 detection are unable to discriminate between mutant and wild-type p53 protein. However, the mutated p53 protein has a longer half-life (4 to 20 h) than wild-type p53 (5 to 20 min), which enables the immunohistochemical detection of the mutated form [33].

Breast carcinoma can be taken as an example for the immunohistochemical determination of p53. The degree of positivity ranged from 15.5% to 54% in 14 breast cancer studies [34]. In positive samples according to 4 different p53 antibodies the frequency of stained cells varied from 29% to 54% depending on the antibody used [35]. These variable results can to some extent be explained by the different patient material, selected or heterogeneous, along with the use of different p53 antibodies recognising different p53 epitopes, and different fixation techniques. The importance of optimal fixation procedures for p53 immunohistochemistry has been highlighted by Silverstrini [36]. Furthermore, the choice of correct cutoff levels for true immunohistochemical p53 positivity has been underlined [36].

In our population-based breast cancer material from 316 patients obtained during a defined time period we discovered a mutation frequency of 21.8% using cDNA-based sequencing [37]. In our comparative study between sequencing and immunohistochemistry using the p53 monoclonal antibody PAb1801 on microwave-retrieved samples we were unable to detect any of the 6 stop codons and we missed 11 of the 13 carcinomas with p53 deletions (Table 2). With reference to prognostic information sequencing was superior; immunohistochemistry revealed similar patterns without reaching the formal significance level of 5% [38]. Our results demonstrate that immunohistochemistry yields both false-negative (23 with negative immunohistochemistry despite mutant p53) and false-positive (19 with positive immunohistochemistry despite wild-type p53) results. As an example of the latter, survival analysis on the complete material identified 19 patients with negative p53 sequencing but with mostly weakly positive immunohistochemistry. These patients had a markedly longer survival than the 43 patients who had tumours which were both immunohistochemically and sequence positive [38].

We have also used higher cutoff levels which impaired the sensitivity (Table 3 and [38]). This procedure did of course increase the specificity and for one pathologist we obtained significance [38]. This type of immunohistochemical subgrouping has, however, been criticised by others [40].

Horne and coworkers [41] in a comparative study explored the p53 antibodies PAb1801, p53-BP-12, D07, and CM1. The best antigen localisation was claimed for PAb1801 and D07. Both these antibodies were used after microwave antigen retrieval which most likely influenced the results [41]. In a series of 245 breast cancer patients included in their comparative immunohistochemical study PAb1801 gave the best prognostic information [41]. These authors obtained a higher frequency of positive samples compared with our study [38,41]. The reasons for the discrepancy between Horne's and our data are not known; one explanation may be the partially different immunohistochemical procedures.

Six p53 antibodies (Bp53-12, PAb1801, D07, PAb240, CM1, and Signet) were used in another study on archival paraffin-embedded colorectal carcinoma material [42]. When used with a "target unmasking fluid" D07 came out best, with a sensitivity and specificity of 67% and 90%, respectively. The positive and negative predictive values were 86% and 75%, respectively [42]. These authors conclude that additional research has to be carried out but also that "immunohistochemistry is valuable for assessing p53 mutations". The complexity of the determination of p53 mutations has recently been analysed [43]. The author claims that sequencing should be the "gold standard". As mentioned above, this technique has some important drawbacks [43].

Table 2. Comparison between immunohistochemical detection of p53 using the monoclonal antibody PAb1801 and sequencing of cDNA

		Point mutations	Deletions		Insertions		Stops	Total
			In frame	*Out of frame*	*In frame*	*Out of frame*		
IHC	+	40	2	0	1	1	0	44
	-	5	3	8	0	1	6	23
	unknown	0	0	0	0	1	1	2
Total		45	5	8	1	3	7	69

From Sjögren et al. J Natl Cancer Inst, 1996; 88: 173-82 [38]

Table 3. Immunohistochemical subclassification based on the PAb1801 monoclonal antibody results; calculated sensitivity and specificity based on the sequencing results

	Immunohistochemistry			
Pathologist	*Negative class*	*Positive class*	**Sensitivity** (%)	**Specificity** (%)
H.N.	0	1, 2, 3, 4, 6, 9	63.8	91.8
	0, 1	2, 3, 4, 6, 9	56.5	95.1
	0, 1, 2	3, 4, 6, 9	49.3	97.1
	0, 1, 2, 3	4, 6, 9	46.4	97.1
	0, 1, 2, 3, 4	6, 9	36.2	97.9
A.L.	0	1, 2, 3, 4, 6, 9	63.8	91.8
	0, 1	2, 3, 4, 6, 9	59.4	93.4
	0, 1, 2	3, 4, 6, 9	44.9	97.1
	0, 1, 2, 3	4, 6, 9	43.4	97.1
	0, 1, 2, 3, 4	6, 9	36.2	98.3

Immunohistochemistry: intensity and extent combined
Intensity: 1: weakly positive cells; 3: strongly positive tumour cells
Extent: 1: less than 1/3 of the tumour cells stained. 3: >2/3 of the tumour cells stained
Results obtained by multiplication of the extent and intensity values
(Adapted from Busch et al, Anticancer Res 1988; 8: 81-8 [39])

The most common molecular biology technique for screening for p53 mutations is the polymerase chain reaction (PCR) combined with single-strand conformation polymorphism (SSCP). Sequencing can thus be performed on samples with altered SSCP patterns. This can either be done directly on DNA or from cDNA. In a review SSCP has been described to detect 71% to 100% of p53 mutations [44]. Using only one glycerol concentration and a fixed temperature we have been unable so far to reproduce such impressive figures [Norberg et al, unpublished]. Our results will most likely improve if other SSCP conditions are tested. If many conditions are required for SSCP one may speculate that direct sequencing of the samples may be more cost-effective, especially since all positive SSCP samples have to be confirmed by sequencing anyway.

Another potentially interesting technique for rapid p53 mutation screening is the constant denaturant gel electrophoresis method [45].

Gumerlock and coworkers [46] have compared the use of RT-PCR-SSCP or DNA-PCR-SSCP on 19 human prostatic carcinomas. Previous examinations of cDNA had revealed 5 wild-type and 14 mutant p53 tumours [46]. These 14 mutants plus one more were identified in the present study. Six of 18 p53 abnormalities (33%) (3 carcinomas had two p53 defects each) were identified by both methods. Ten of the 18 p53 abnormalities were only demonstrated with the RT-PCR-SSCP method as against 2 of the 18 with the DNA-PCR-SSCP method. The confidence intervals for these figures are of course very wide and must therefore be interpreted with caution. These data indicate that RNA as a source may in some instances be preferable to DNA. The explanation for the better yield using RNA may be selectively enhanced RNA levels in the carcinoma cells versus normal stroma cells. However, the use of DNA has clear advantages as it gives access to the large tumour banks of paraffin-embedded material at all pathology institutions. It will be important to obtain detailed pathology reports on all these samples in order to be able to relate the molecular biology findings to classic histopathology. However, clinical data on type of therapy and outcome data for each individual patient will of course be the cornerstone of and prerequisite for this type of studies.

p53 and prognosis

Mutations of the p53 gene is the most common genetic abnormality in human cancer. The figures must be interpreted with some caution because the majority of studies have used positive immunohistochemistry as a surrogate endpoint for true mutation. The frequency of p53 mutations varies from only a few percent in testicular teratomas and Wilms' tumours to more than 50% in lung and colon carcinoma [25,47]. p53 mutations have been reported to be associated with a worse prognosis for patients with bladder, colon, oesophageal, gastric, non-small cell lung, ovarian, and prostate carcinoma and soft tissue sarcomas [22,48-55].

With reference to breast carcinoma several studies have demonstrated that mutant p53 or enhanced p53 protein levels result in a significantly worse prognosis [37,56-60]. We analysed the p53 status using both cDNA sequencing and immunohistochemistry in breast carcinoma material of 316 patients collected from 1987 to 1989 [37,38]. The material was consecutive and derived from a defined geographical region; it included all tumours from which we had frozen material, which was the standard procedure since 1978. However, patients with too small breast cancers were not included because all material had been used for routine histopathological examination. The median follow-up was 57 months, with a maximum of 87 months [38].

The Uppsala study revealed a significantly worse survival for patients with p53 mutations both in univariate and multivariate analysis in the total material and for node-positive patients, but not for the node-negative subgroup. The same trends were observed using the monoclonal antibody PAb1801, but the differences did not reach statistical significance [38]. These findings are partly contradictory to the study performed by Elledge and coworkers [58], who demonstrated prognostic value also for node-negative patients using immunohistochemistry. The same group reported that the combination of the p53 antibodies PAb240 and PAb1801 gave the best discriminative result for node-negative breast cancers [61]. In the same article these authors compared the immunohistochemistry results for the different antibodies singly or in combination (PAb1801/PAb240, PAb240, PAb1801, 421, CM1, BP53-12) and SSCP, which gave discordant outcomes [61].

p53 mutation locations with reference to prognosis

The locations of the mutations showed a difference between node-positive and node-negative patients with respect to mutations located within the evolutionarily conserved regions [37]. The node-positive patients tended to have more mutations in the evolutionarily conserved regions II and V [37]. These patients had a significantly worse relapse-free, breast cancer-corrected and overall survival than patients with p53 mutations located in the conserved regions III and IV, or outside the evolutionarily conserved regions (Fig. 2). The lymph node-negative patients tended to have relatively more p53 mutations within the evolutionarily conserved regions III and IV than node-positive patients. Furthermore, the relapse-free, breast cancer-corrected and total survival were almost similar for patients without p53 mutations (Fig. 2). Of course these results should be interpreted with great caution because they are based on subgroup analysis of small patient numbers and on retrospective material, but the data indicate fairly strongly that the site of mutation may be very important. This is further underlined by findings by Børresen and coworkers [62], who demonstrated in breast cancer material that mutations located in the zinc binding domains L2 and L3 were associated with a worse prognosis. One may thus speculate that certain mutations are "silent", although they are missense mutations, leaving the p53 protein "intact" with respect to its function. The opposite may be true for other mutations, e.g. p53 alterations within certain loca-

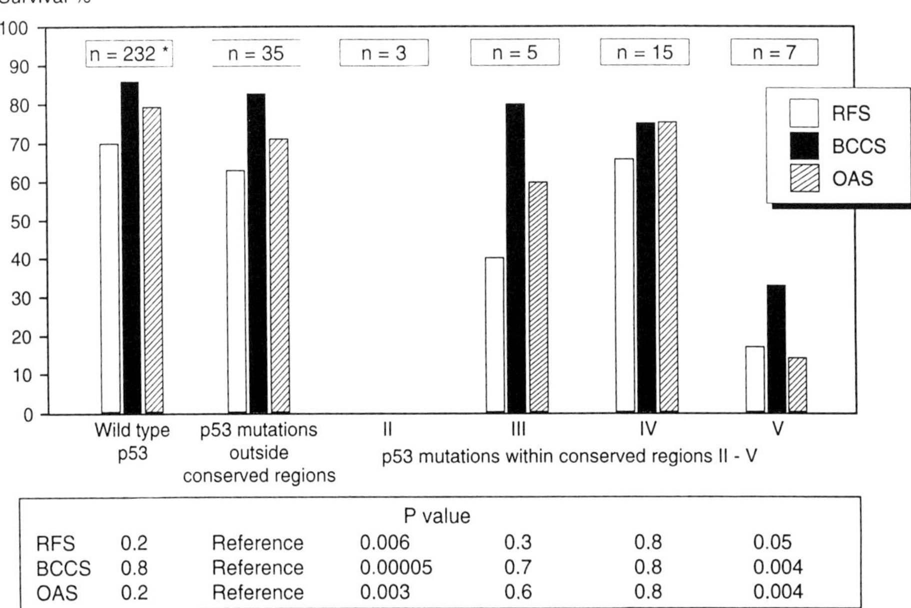

	P value				
RFS	0.2	Reference	0.006	0.3	0.8	0.05
BCCS	0.8	Reference	0.00005	0.7	0.8	0.004
OAS	0.2	Reference	0.003	0.6	0.8	0.004

* 233 patients were available for BCCS and OAS

Fig. 2. The outcome for 316 breast cancer patients operated on from 1987 to 1989 representing a population-based cohort. The analysis was based on 298 patients as we lacked information on node status in 13 patients and on survival in 1, while p53 sequences were incomplete for 4 patients [37]. p53 mutation locations outside or within the evolutionarily conserved regions (II to V) together with tumours containing wild-type p53 are outlined in relation to prognosis. RFS: Relapse-free survival; BCCS: Breast cancer-corrected survival; OAS: Overall survival.
From Bergh et al, Nature Med, 1995; 10: 1029-34 [37]

tions such as the evolutionarily conserved regions II and V or the L2 and L3 domains. p53 determination techniques other than sequencing will not provide this type of detailed information relevant to prognosis. Further studies of the p53 mutation locations may provide a rational explanation of our findings and those of other authors with reference to the predictive value in relation to used therapeutic agents.

p53 may thus be added to the list of prognostic factors for a wide range of human cancers. The clinical use of p53 as a prognostic factor will not be generally accepted until it has been demonstrated to be independent of confounding factors in multivariate analyses. Furthermore, the best way to test its validity is to perform a prospective and controlled study.

p53 as a predictive factor

Preclinical studies but now also retrospective clinical studies have revealed that tumours containing mutant p53 show a poorer response to the majority of currently used cytotoxic compounds, radiation and tamoxifen [37,63-72]. Antimitotic and tubulin interfering agents like docetaxel and paclitaxel were among the few examples of cytostatics shown to be active even in p53 mutated cells [72]. Furthermore, the promoter for the multidrug resistance gene has been described to be activated by ras and p53 [73]. This underlines that, besides altered p53-directed apoptosis, other mechanisms are directly or indirectly involved in resistance to cytostatics [74-77].

Lymph node-positive patients in the Uppsala series who received adjuvant tamoxifen in combination with local/locoregional radiotherapy, mostly post-menopausal women, had a significantly worse prognosis if they had breast carcinomas with p53 mutations compared with the subgroup of patients with wild-type p53 [37]. Similar trends were observed for the corresponding premenopausal group receiving adjuvant polychemotherapy, mostly cyclophosphamide, methotrexate and 5-fluorouracil, in combination with local/locoregional radiotherapy. However, in this limited patient number this potential difference did not reach formal statistical significance [37].

We have also studied the subgroup of patients with lymph node-negative disease who were treated either with surgery and local or locoregional radiotherapy or surgery without postoperative radiation [78]. The 168 patients with wild-type p53 showed only a slight trend in favour of postoperative radiation with reference to relapse-free, breast cancer-corrected and total survival. On the other hand, in the retrospective subanalysis of the 30 patients with mutant tumour p53, postoperative radiotherapy resulted in a significant improvement in relapse-free, breast cancer-corrected and overall survival. Our findings in this retrospective subgroup analysis of non-randomised material were essentially sustained in the multivariate analysis [78]. A very recent retrospective study on 635 patients using immunohistochemistry demonstrated a statistically significantly increased local control by radiotherapy in patients with p53 protein alterations [79]. Of course, these observations must be interpreted with caution and serve mainly to generate hypotheses for further studies, preferably in the form of prospective trials using randomisation based on the p53 status.

The complexity of the relationship between p53 status and response to radiotherapy is underlined by the partially contradictory findings in two studies regarding the ability of p53 to induce apoptosis in the wild-type and mutated condition [65,80].

The increased local control in the two studies mainly in patients with p53 alterations will be potentially important information for the discussion regarding which patients have benefit from postoperative radiotherapy, but the other two findings were slightly surprising since a recent meta-analysis was unable to detect any survival benefit from postoperative radiation [81]. The findings of the large EBCTCG overview [81] may be explained by the fact that postoperative radiation is associated with increased cardiovascular mortality for left-sided breast carcinomas. However, there are indications of survival benefits for certain subgroups of patients receiving postoperative radiotherapy [82]. Theoretically, if postoperative radiation is given with heart-sparing techniques certain subgroups may have potential survival benefits. One may speculate that certain p53 mutation locations in the group of node-negative breast carcinomas may result in preserved p53 function resulting in apoptosis induced by radiation.

Future prospects

p53 has been demonstrated to be an important prognostic factor for several malignancies and it is a potentially important predictive factor for breast cancer. As indicated above the gene is a key regulator of essential cellular processes. The latter facts combined with its predictive value are major reasons why gene therapy studies with p53 have been initiated on patients with demonstrated p53 abnormalities in their tumours [14,83]. A recent clinical study using a retroviral vector containing wild-type p53 in nine patients with non-small cell lung cancer bearing p53 mutations demonstrated tumour regression in three patients and stable disease in another three [84]. However, all patients finally progressed but this report further underlines the powerful potential of p53 gene therapy.

The precise and correct description and diagnosis of the p53 status before and after gene therapy with p53 is of fundamental importance. Following these initial studies focusing on the p53 gene further investigations will involve a detailed analysis of p53 and its downstream mediators. This may enable us to identify multiple mechanisms of the pathological behaviour in cancer cells versus normal cells with homeostasis in those regulatory pathways. The diagnosis of these disturbances should be as precise as possible. This, in turn, may enable us to develop even further selective strategies for the normalisation of abnormalities in p53 function and that of its downstream mediators. However, for the common solid tumours this tailored approach will most likely be complicated by heterogeneity in the regulatory pathways.

Acknowledgements

This study has been supported by grants from the Swedish Cancer Society, Lions research fund at Akademiska sjukhuset, the "ALF-foundation" at Akademiska sjukhuset and Pharmacia Biotech. Many thanks to Drs Mats Inganäs and Sigrid Sjögren for their help with the material and for their suggestions. The secretarial assistance of Marléne Forslund is very much appreciated.

References

1   Bonadonna G, Rossi A, Valagussa P, Banfi A, Veronesi U. The CMF program for operable breast cancer cancer with positive nodes. Cancer 1977; 39: 2904-15
2   Early Breast Cancer Trialists' Collaborative Group. Systemic treatment of early breast cancer by hormonal, cytotoxic, or immune therapy. Lancet 1992; 339:1-15, 71-85
3   Nyström L, Rutqvist LE, Wall S et al. Breast cancer screening with mammography: Overview of Swedish randomised trials. Lancet 1993; 341: 973-8
4   Sakr WA, Haas GP, Gassin BF, Pontes JE, Crissman JD. The frequency of carcinoma and intraepithelial neoplasia of the prostate in young male patients. J Urol 1993; 150: 379-85
5   Campbell FC, Blamey RW, Elston CW et al. Quantitative oestradiol receptor values in primary breast cancer and response of metastases to endocrine therapy. Lancet 1981; 2: 1317-9
6   Muss HB, Thor AD, Berry DA et al. c-erbB-2 expression and response to adjuvant therapy in women with node-positive early breast cancer. N Engl J Med 1994; 330: 1260-6
7   Stål O, Sullivan S, Wingren S et al. c-erbB-2 expression and benefit from adjuvant chemotherapy and radiotherapy of breast cancer. Eur J Cancer 1995; 31A: 2185-90
8   Allred DC, Clark GM, Tandon AK et al. HER-2/neu in node-negative breast cancer: prognostic significance of overexpression influenced by the presence of in situ carcinoma. J Clin Oncol 1992; 10: 599-605
9   Gusterson BA, Belber RD, Goldhirsch A et al. Prognostic importance of c-erbB-2 expression in breast cancer. J Clin Oncol 1992; 10: 1049-56
10 Klijn JGM, Berns EMJJ, Foekens JA. Prognostic factors and response to therapy in breast cancer. Cancer Surveys 1993; 18: 165-98
11 Carlomagno C, Perrone F, Gallo C et al. c-erbB2 overexpression decreases the benefit of adjuvant tamoxifen in early -stage breast cancer without axillary lymph node metastases. J Clin Oncol 1996; 14: 2702-8
12 Kastan MB. The p53 tumor suppressor gene. Advances in Oncology 1996; 12: 3-7
13 Lane D. p53, guardian of the genome. Nature 1992; 358: 15-6
14 Harris CC. Structure and function of the p53 tumor suppressor gene: Clues for rational cancer therapeutic strategies. J Natl Cancer Inst 1996; 88: 1442-55
15 Mcbride OW, Merry D, Givol D. The gene for human p53 cellular tumor antigene is located on chromosome 17 short arm (17p13). Proc Natl Acad Sci USA 1986; 83: 130-4
16 Miller C, Mohandas T, Wolf D, Prokocimer M, Rotter V, Koeffler HP. Human p53 localized to short arm of chromosome 17. Nature 1986; 319: 783-4
17 Soussi T, Caron de Fromentel C, May P. Structural aspects of the p53 protein in relation to gene evolution. Oncogene 1990; 5: 945-52
18 Cho Y, Gorina S, Jeffery P, Pavletich N. Crystal structure of a p53 tumor suppressor-DNA complex: Understanding tumorigenic mutations. Science 1994; 265: 346-55
19 Gorina S, Pavletich NP. Structure of the p53 tumor suppressor bound to the ankyrin and SH3 domains of 53BP2. Science 1996; 274: 1001-5
20 Kussie PH, Gorina S, Marechal V et al. Structure of the MDM2 oncoprotein bound to the p53 tumor suppressor transactivation domain. Science 1996; 274: 948-53
21 Vogelstein B, Kinzler KW. p53 function and dysfunction. Cell 1992; 70: 523-6
22 Chang F, Syrjänen S, Syrjänen K. Implications of the p53 tumor-suppressor gene in clinical oncology. J Clin Oncol 1995; 13: 1009-22
23 Stinchcomb DT. Constraining the cell cycle: Regulating cell division and differentiation by gene therapy. Nature Medicine 1995; 1: 1004-6
24 Norberg T, Jansson T, Sjögren S et al. Overview on human breast cancer with focus on prognostic and predictive factors with special attention on the tumour suppressor gene p53. Acta Oncol1996; 35 (suppl 5): 96-102

25 Velculescu VE, El-Deiry WS. Biological and clinical importance of the p53 tumor suppressor gene. Clin Chem 1996; 42: 858-68
26 Malkin D, Li FP, Strong LC et al. Germ line p53 mutations in a familial syndrome of breast cancer, sarcomas, and other neoplasms. Science 1990; 250: 1233-8
27 Srivastava S, Zou ZQ, Pirollo K, Blattner W, Chang EH. Germ-line transmission of a mutated p53 gene in a cancer-prone family with Li-Fraumeni syndrome. Nature 1990; 348: 747-9
28 Donehower LA, Harvey M, Slagle BL et al. Mice deficient for p53 are developmentally normal but susceptible to spontaneous tumours. Nature 1992; 356: 215-21
29 Kastan MB, Zhan Q, el-Deiry WS et al. A mammalian cell cycle checkpoint pathway utilizing p53 and GADD45 is defective in ataxia-telangiectasia. Cell 1992; 71: 587-97
30 Canman CE, Wolff AC, Chen C et al. The p53-dependent G1 cell cycle checkpoint pathway and ataxia-telangiectasia. Cancer Res 1994; 54: 5054-8
31 Savitsky K, Bar-Shira A, Gilad S et al. A single ataxia telangiectasia gene with a product similar to PI-3 kinase. Science 1995; 268: 1749-53
32 Yin C, Knudson M, Korsmeyer SJ, Van Dyke T. Bax suppresses and stimulates apoptosis in vivo. Nature 1997; 385: 637-40
33 Hesketh R. Tumour suppressor genes, p53. In: The oncogene handbook. London: Academic Press Ltd 1994; 536-53
34 Bhargava V, Thor A, Deng G et al. The association of p53 immunopositivity with tumor proliferation and other prognostic indicators in breast cancer. Modern Pathol 1994; 7: 361-8
35 Jacquemier J, Moles JP, Pennault-Llorca F et al. p53 immunohistochemical analysis in breast cancer with four monoclonal antibodies: comparison of staining and PCR-SSCP results. Br J Cancer 1994; 69: 846-52
36 Silvestrini R. The p53 gene in breast cancer: Prognostic value of complementary DNA sequencing versus immunohistochemistry. J Natl Cancer Inst 1996; 88: 1499
37 Bergh J, Norberg T, Sjögren S, Lindgren A, Holmberg L. Complete sequencing of the p53 gene provides prognostic information in breast cancer patients, particularly in relation to adjuvant systemic therapy and radiotherapy. Nature Medicine 1995; 1: 1029-34
38 Sjögren S, Inganäs M, Norberg T et al. The p53 gene in breast cancer: Prognostic value of complementary DNA sequencing versus immunohistochemistry. J Natl Cancer Inst 1996; 88: 173-82
39 Busch C, Malmström PO, Norlén BJ et al. A grading system for the immunostaining of A, B and H blood group isoantigens in bladder carcinoma. Anticancer Res 1988; 8: 81-8
40 Kay EW, Walsh CJ, Cassidy M, Curran B, Leader M. C-erbB-2 immunostaining: problems with interpretation. J Clin Pathol 1994; 47: 816-22
41 Horne GM, Anderson JJ, Tiniakos DG et al. p53 protein as a prognostic indicator in breast carcinoma: a comparison of four antibodies for immunohistochemistry. Br J Cancer 1996; 73: 29-35
42 Baas IO, Mulder JW, Offerhaus GJ, Vogelstein B, Hamilton SR. An evaluation of six antibodies for immunohistochemistry of mutant p53 gene product in archival colorectal neoplasms. J Pathol 1994; 172: 5-12
43 Elledge RM. Assessing p53 status in breast cancer prognosis: Where should you put the thermometer if you think your p53 is sick? J Natl Cancer Inst 1996; 88: 141-3
44 Hayashi K, Yandell DW. How sensitive is PCR-SSCP? Hum Mutat 1993; 2: 338-46
45 Børresen A-L, Hovig E, Smith-Sørensen B et al. Constant denaturant gel electrophoresis as rapid screening technique for p53 mutations. Proc Natl Acad Sci USA 1991; 88: 8405-9
46 Gumerlock PH, Chi S-G, Shi X-B et al. The Cooperative Prostate Network. p53 abnormalities in primary prostate cancer: Single-strand conformation polymorphism analysis of complementary DNA in comparison with genomic DNA. J Natl Cancer Inst 1997; 89: 66-71

47 Greenblatt MS, Bennett WP, Hollstein M, Harris, CC. Mutations in the p53 tumor suppressor gene: Clues to cancer etiology and molecular pathogenesis. Cancer Res 1994; 54: 4855-78

48 Sarkis AS, Dalbagni G, Cordon-Cardo C et al. Nuclear overexpression of p53 protein in transitional cell bladder carcinoma: A marker for disease progression. J Natl Cancer Inst 1993; 85: 53-9

49 Remvikos Y, Tominaga O, Hammel P et al. Increased p53 protein content of colorectal tumours correlates with poor survival. Br J Cancer 1992; 66: 758-64

50 Starzynska T, Bromley M, Ghosh A, Stern PL. Prognostic significance of p53 overexpression in gastric and colorectal carcinoma. Br J Cancer 1992; 66: 558-62

51 Martin HM, Filipe MI, Morris RW, Lane DP, Silvestre F. p53 expression and prognosis in gastric carcinoma. Int J Cancer 1992; 50: 859-62

52 Mitsudomi T, Oyama T, Kusano T, Osaki T, Nakanishi R, Shirakusa T. Mutations of the p53 gene as a predictor of poor prognosis in patients with non-small-cell lung cancer. J Natl Cancer Inst 1993; 85: 2018-23

53 Bosari S, Viale G, Radaelli U, Bossi P, Bonoldi E, Coggi G. p53 accumulation in ovarian carcinoma and its prognostic implications. Hum Pathol 1993; 24: 1175-9

54 Visakorpi T, Kallioniemi OP, Heikkinen A, Koivula T, Isola J. Small subgroup of aggressive, highly proliferative prostatic carcinomas defined by p53 accumulation. J Natl Cancer Inst 1992; 84: 883-7

55 Drobnjak M, Latres E, Pollack D et al. Prognostic implications of p53 nuclear overexpression and high proliferation index of Ki-67 in adult soft-tissue sarcomas. J Natl Cancer Inst 1994; 86: 549-54

56 Thor A, Moore II D, Edgerton S et al. Accumulation of p53 tumor suppressor gene protein: An independent marker of prognosis in breast cancers. J Natl Cancer Inst 1992; 84: 845-55

57 Andersen TI, Holm R, Nesland JM, Heimdal KR, Ottestad L, Børresen A-L. Prognostic significance of TP53 alterations in breast carcinoma Br J Cancer 1993; 68: 540-8

58 Elledge R, Fuqua S, Clark G, Pujol P, Allred D, McGuire W. Prognostic significance of p53 gene alterations in node-negative breast cancer. Br Cancer Res Treat 1993; 26: 225-35

59 Thorlacius S, Børresen A, Eyfjörd J. Somatic p53 mutations in human breast carcinomas in an Icelandic population: A prognostic factor. Cancer Res 1993; 53: 1637-41

60 Borg Å, Lennerstrand J, Stemark-Askmalm M et al. Prognostic significance of p53 overexpression in primary breast cancer; a novel luminometric immunoassay applicable on steroid receptor cytosols. Br J Cancer 1995; 71: 1013-7

61 Elledge R, Clark G, Fuqua S, Yu Y-Y, Allred D. p53 protein accumulation detected by five different antibodies: Relationship to prognosis and heat shock protein 70 in breast cancer. Cancer Res 1994; 54: 3752-7

62 Børresen AL, Andersen TI, Eyfjord JE et al. TP53 mutations and breast cancer prognosis: particularly poor survival rates for cases with mutations in the zinc-binding domains. Genes Chromosom Cancer 1995; 14: 71-5

63 Clarke AR, Purdie CA, Harrison DJ et al. Thymocyte apoptosis induced by p53-dependent and independent pathways. Nature 1993; 362: 849-52

64 Lowe S, Ruley H, Jacks T, Housman D. p53-dependent apoptosis modulates the cytotoxicity of anticancer agents. Cells 1993; 74: 957-67

65 O'Connor P, Jackman J, Jondle D, Bhatia K, Magrath I, Kohn K. Role of the p53 tumor suppressor gene in cell cycle arrest and radiosensitivity of Burkitt's lymphoma cell lines. Cancer Res 1993; 53: 4776-80

66 Fan S, El-Deiry WS, Bae I et al. p53 gene mutations are associated with decreased sensitivity of human lymphoma cells to DNA damaging agents. Cancer Res 1994; 54: 5824-30

50   J. Bergh

67   Lim J, Bhimani R, Frenkel K, Troll W. The chemopreventive agent tamoxifen causes apoptosis. Proc Annu Meet Am Assoc Cancer Res 1994, abstract 3693

68   Lowe S, Bodis S, McClatchey A et al. p53 status and the efficacy of cancer therapy in vivo. Science 1994; 266: 807-10

69   Wattel E, Preudhomme C, Hecquet B et al. p53 mutations are associated with resistance to chemotherapy and short survival in hematologic malignancies. Blood 1994; 84: 3148-57

70   Righetti SC, Della Torre G, Polotti S et al. A comparative study of p53 gene mutations, protein accumulation, and response to cisplatin-based chemotherapy in advanced ovarian carcinoma. Cancer Res 1996; 56: 689-93

71   Aas T, Børresen A-L, Geisler S et al. Specific p53 mutations are associated with de novo resistance to doxorubicin in breast cancer patients. Nature Med 1996; 2: 811-4

72   Weinstein JN, Myers TG, O'Connor PM. An information-intensive approach to the molecular pharmacology of cancer. Science 1997; 275: 343-9

73   Chin KV, Ueda K, Pastan I, Gottesman MM. Modulation of activity of the promoter of the human MDR1 gene by Ras and p53. Science 1992; 255: 459-62

74   Cole SPC, Bhardwaj G, Gerlach JH et al. Overexpression of a transporter gene in a multidrug-resistant human lung cancer cell line. Science 1992; 258: 1650-4

75   Chin KV, Pastan I, Gottesman MM. Function and regulation of the human multidrug resistance gene. Adv Cancer Res 1993; 60: 157-80

76   Watt PM, Hickson ID. Structure and function of type II DNA topoisomerases. Biochem J 1994; 303: 681-95

77   de la Torre M. Drug resistance associated proteins in human breast cancer. Acta Universitatis Upsaliensis 1994; 514: 1-54

78   Jansson T, Inganäs M, Sjögren S et al. p53 status predicts survival in breast cancer patients treated with or without postoperative radiotherapy: A novel hypothesis based on clinical findings. J Clin Oncol 1995; 13: 2745-51

79   Bergh J. Time for integration of predictive factors for selection of breast cancer patients who need postoperative radiation. J Natl Cancer Inst 1997; 89: 605-7

80   Xia F, Wang X, Wang Y-H. Altered p53 status correlates with differences in sensitivity to radiation-induced mutation and apoptosis in two closely related human lymphoblast lines. Cancer Res 1995; 55: 12-5

81   Early Breast Cancer Trialists' Collaborative Group. Effects of radiotherapy and surgery in early breast cancer. An overview of the randomized trials. N Engl J Med 1995; 333: 1444-55

82   Cuzick J, Stewart H, Rutqvist L et al. Cause-specific mortality in long-term survivors of breast cancer who participated in trials of radiotherapy. J Clin Oncol 1994; 12: 447-53

83   Roth JA, Cristiano RJ. Gene therapy: What have we done and where are we going. J Natl Cancer Inst 1997; 89: 21-39

84   Roth JA, Nguyen D, Lawrence DD et al. Retrovirus-mediated wild-type p53 gene transfer to tumors of patients with lung cancer. Nature Med 1996; 2: 985-91

ESO Scientific Updates, Vol. 1
Prognostic and Predictive Value of p53
J.G.M. Klijn, editor
© 1997 Elsevier Science B.V. All rights reserved

Prognostic and Predictive Significance of p53 Protein Accumulation in Human Primary Breast Cancer Analysed with a Luminometric Immunoassay (LIA) on Tumour Cytosols

Els M.J.J. Berns, John A. Foekens and Jan G.M. Klijn

Division of Endocrine Oncology of the Department of Medical Oncology, Rotterdam Cancer Institute (Daniel den Hoed Kliniek)/University Hospital Rotterdam, The Netherlands

Introduction

The human tumour suppressor gene p53 (also known as TP53) is located on chromosome band 17p13.1. It consists of 11 separate exons, of which the first one is non-coding, and the resulting protein product of 393 amino acids has a molecular weight of 53 kDa [1]. This nuclear phosphoprotein can function as a transcription factor and *in vitro* studies suggest that oligomerization of wild-type p53 is necessary for sequence-specific DNA binding [2]. p53 is the most frequently mutated gene in human tumours, and reintroduction of the gene into transformed cells can either induce growth arrest [3] or apoptosis [4].

   p53 has been implicated in the regulation of normal cell growth and division, genomic stability, DNA repair, senescence and apoptosis (see [5,6] for review). Thus p53 functions as the "guardian of the genome" and the normal function of p53 is to effect cell cycle arrest at the G1 and G2 checkpoints in response to DNA damage [7-9]. The regulation of p53 expression in response to DNA damage is not completely understood. p53 binds to damaged DNA in a non-specific fashion via its C-terminal 75 amino acids [10]. After DNA damage the intracellular levels of wild-type p53 rise and induce the transcription of effector genes such as p21$^{WAF/CIPI/SDI1}$ and GADD45 (growth arrest on DNA damage) as shown in Figure 1. p21 inactivates a broad spectrum of G1 and G2 cyclin-cyclin dependent kinases (cdk) complexes, including cdk-2 and 4, which results in a G1/S phase arrest of the cell cycle and allows for extra repair time [11,12]. Both GADD45 and p21 bind to the proliferating cell nuclear antigen (PCNA), which is an essential accessory factor to the DNA polymerase-∂. This

Address for correspondence: E.M.J.J. Berns, Division of Endocrine Oncology, Rotterdam Cancer Institute (Daniel den Hoed Kliniek)/University Hospital Rotterdam, P.O. Box 5201, 3008 AE Rotterdam, The Netherlands. Tel: +31-10-4391725, Fax: +31-10-4232964, e-mail: berns@bidh.azr.nl

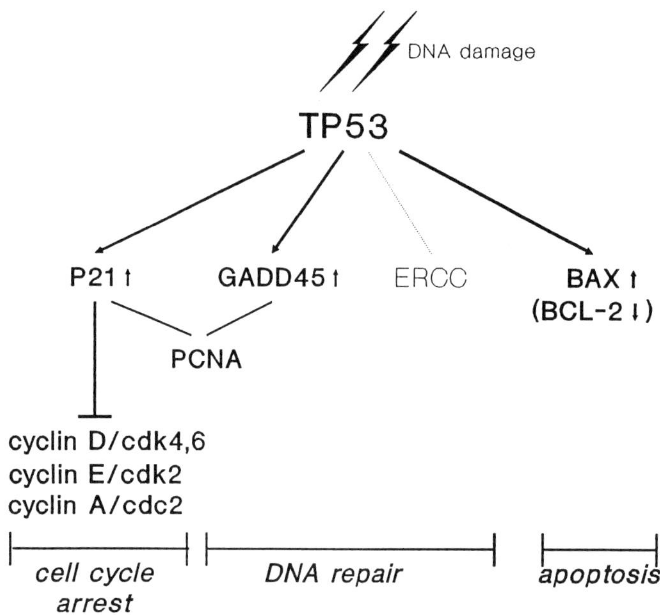

Fig. 1. The current model of p53 function postulates that p53 senses DNA damage and arrests the cell cycle in either G1 or G2 phase, so that DNA repair can take place (see text for explanation). For cells that have sustained irreparable DNA damage, apoptosis is the means to eliminate the cells through wild-type p53 [3,14,33]. However, the *mutated* form of p53 is not able to accomplish this.

latter enzyme is required for leading strand replication and DNA repair, and is an essential cofactor for replicative DNA synthesis [13]. Thus, binding of p21 or GADD45 to PCNA results in redistribution of PCNA from sites of DNA replication to sites of DNA damage. p53 may also bind to ERCC3, which is implicated in excision repair [12]. In addition p53 has been found to trigger apoptosis [14, 15] and current data show that wild-type p53 can induce apoptosis by upregulation of bax *in vitro* and *in vivo* (16) and down-regulation of bcl-2, a suppressor of apoptosis. Halder et al. [17] provided evidence that p53 protein expression is inversely correlated with bcl-2 protein expression in breast cancer cell lines.

Inactivation of p53 is one of the most common molecular genetic events described so far in the development of cancer. This inactivation may occur by binding of the p53 protein to viral transforming proteins simian virus 40 (SV40) large T antigen, adenovirus E1B and E6 gene product of human papillomavirus, or by binding to the cellular oncogene product of the murine double minute-2 (mdm-2) protein, which is transactivated by p53, or to heat shock protein (hsp) 70, which all neutralise its activity. Another way to inactivate p53 gene function is through gene mutation (see [18] for review) and since the remaining p53 allele is commonly deleted or in some cases affected by an independent point mutation, all wild-type p53 activity will be eliminated.

p53 gene mutation is the most prevalent gene alteration described so far in human primary breast cancer. Several molecular biological techniques are used to analyse mutations in the p53 gene. These include polymerase chain reaction (PCR) driven single-strand conformation analysis (SSCA), denaturing gradient gel electrophoresis (DGGE), constant denaturant gel electrophoresis (CDGE) and sequence analyses. The mutations are mostly missense, which result in a stably expressed conformationally altered protein with an increased half-life. The ensuing accumulation is detectable by immunological techniques such as immunohistochemistry, ELISA, and Western blotting [19,20]. The recently developed luminometric immunoassay, LIA [21], allows a rapid analysis of p53 protein accumulation in large (retrospective) series of primary breast tumour cytosols which are routinely prepared for steroid hormone receptor analysis.

In the present analysis on a large series of breast tumour cytosols we aimed to determine whether p53 protein accumulation, as determined by LIA, was associated with i) patient or tumour characteristics and prognosis; ii) response to first-line tamoxifen therapy; and iii) response to first-line polychemotherapy.

Methods

Tumours and patients

In the studies reported here only primary breast tumour specimens, collected between 1978-1991 and used for routine steroid hormone receptor analysis, from patients with known follow-up were included. These specimens were stored in liquid nitrogen. The samples were pulverised in the frozen state and homogenised in a phosphate buffer according to procedures recommended by the EORTC for the preparation of cytosols for receptor (ER and PgR) measurement (EORTC Breast Cancer Cooperative Group [22]). Receptors were measured by ligand binding assay or with enzyme immunoassays [23]. All patients had primary invasive breast cancer with no signs of distant metastasis at the time of surgery. Detailed information on patient and tumour characteristics are given in the "Results" section for each subset analysed.

Luminometric immunoassay

The p53 protein levels of the breast tumour cytosols were measured with a quantitative luminometric immunoassay (LIA; AB Sangtec Medical, Bromma, Sweden), described elsewhere [21,24]. The LIA is based on a combination of two monoclonal antibodies, 1801 and DO1, which detect both wild-type and mutant p53 protein in a sandwich-type assay. The monoclonal antibody 1801, which is immobilised onto a solid phase (the tube), is used for catching. Monoclonal antibody DO1, labelled with a chemiluminescent compound (amino-butyl-ethyl-isoluminol: ABEI), is used for detection. The immunoassay was performed by incubating either 100 µl of p53 standard (range: 0-80 ng/ml), controls or tumour cytosols, together with 100 µl of the ABEI-conjugate in pre-coated tubes. After incubation for 18 hours at room temperature, unbound reagents were removed by washing the tubes three times with 2 ml 0.9% sodium chloride. The chemiluminescent reaction was initiated by the sequential addition of 300 µl alkaline hydrogen peroxide and 300 µl catalyst (microperoxidase) solution, immediately followed by measurement of the chemiluminescent counts in a luminometer. The p53 protein contents of the samples were determined from the standard curve, plotting the chemiluminescent response (in relative light units: RLU) against the standard concentrations of the p53 protein. The detection limit is approximately 0.01 ng p53 per ml sample. The concentration of p53 protein in the tumour cytosols is expressed as ng/mg cytosolic protein (the protein concentration of all samples was brought to 0.5 mg/ml cytosol, with kit diluent buffer).

Statistical analysis

The relationships between p53 protein levels and patient and tumour characteristics were studied with non-parametric tests: the Wilcoxon test (menopausal status, tumour size, ER, PgR), the Kruskall-Wallis test including a Wilcoxon-type test for trend for ordered variables (nodal status) and the Spearman rank correlation for continuous variables. Relapse-free survival probabilities were calculated by the actuarial method of Kaplan and Meier [25]. The Cox proportional hazard model was used for uni- and multivariate survival analyses.

Results and discussion

p53 levels, patient and tumour characteristics and prognosis

The p53-LIA was performed on approximately 1500 primary breast tumour cytosols. Fifteen separate experiments were required to obtain all results. In each experiment the kit controls ("low" and "high"), a "reference" preparation and a tumour "cytosol pool" were included. The assay results were highly reproducible with between-assay variations of these four controls ranging from 5.6% to 11.2%. The p53 protein values in cytosols ranged between 0 and 154 ng/mg cytosolic protein (with a median level of 0.20 ng/mg protein).

The median age of the patients was 56 years (range: 24-89 years). Forty-one percent of the patients were premenopausal, 26% had no involved lymph nodes, and 41% of the tumours were smaller than 2 cm (T1). Of these patients 23% received adjuvant treatment. The median follow-up of patients alive was 66 months. During follow-up 46% of the patients had a relapse and 34% died. With regard to patient and tumour characteristics there were no significant relationships between p53 protein levels and menopausal status, nodal status or tumour size (Fig. 2). The Spearman rank correlation coefficient between the lev-

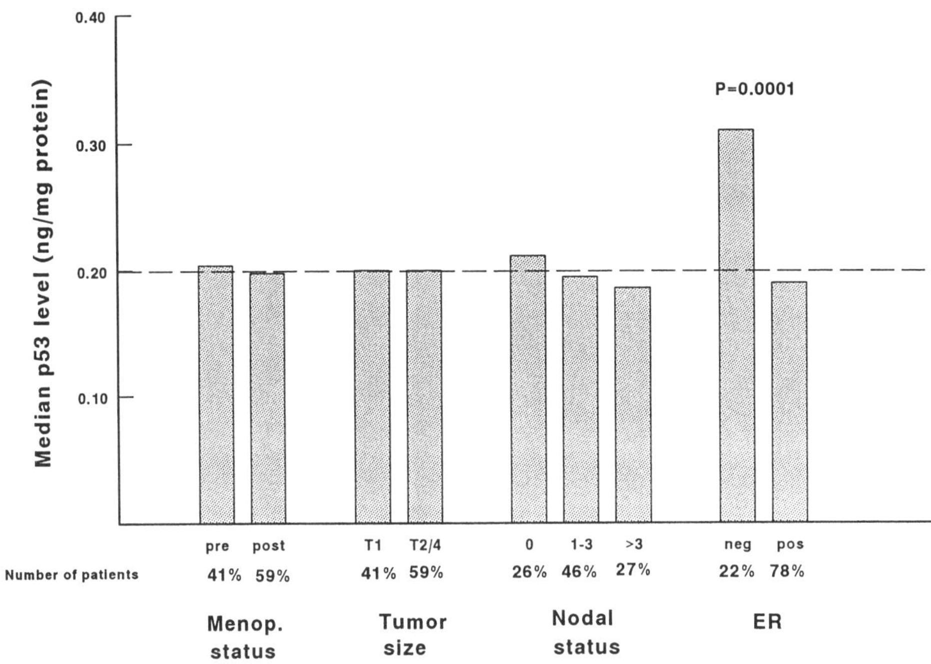

Fig. 2. Relationship of p53 with patient and tumour characteristics.

els of p53 with ER was -0.06 (not significant). In ER-negative tumours median p53 protein levels were significantly higher than in ER-positive tumours (p= 0.0001, see Fig. 2). In Cox's univariate regression analysis using dichotomised (at the median level) or logarithmically transformed values, high p53 levels were related to a shorter relapse-free (RFS) and overall survival (p=0.01).

We have used log transformation to create a more symmetrical distribution of the factor, shrunk at 1%, and regression analysis was applied next. The analysis was applied with relapse-free survival as the endpoint for all tumour samples, and 0.38 ng/mg protein was chosen as the cutoff point to discriminate between accumulated p53 (high) protein (34%) and low p53 protein levels (66%). This prevalence is comparable with the p53 protein accumulation of 30% and 28% observed in smaller series of breast tumours studied by Borg et al. [21] and by our group [24], respectively. Moreover, this is well in line with the percentage of p53 gene alterations or p53 protein overexpression observed in 14-52% of 3000 human breast tumours using either molecular or immunological techniques (see [26] for review). In univariate analysis p53 protein accumulation was significantly associated with an increased relapse rate (p=0.001), and this association seems more prominent during the first 3 years (Fig. 3). In a multivariate analysis for relapse-free survival, including age, menopausal status, tumour size, nodal status and steroid hormone receptor status, p53 protein accumulation (analysed as a dichotomized variable) was an independent factor for predict-

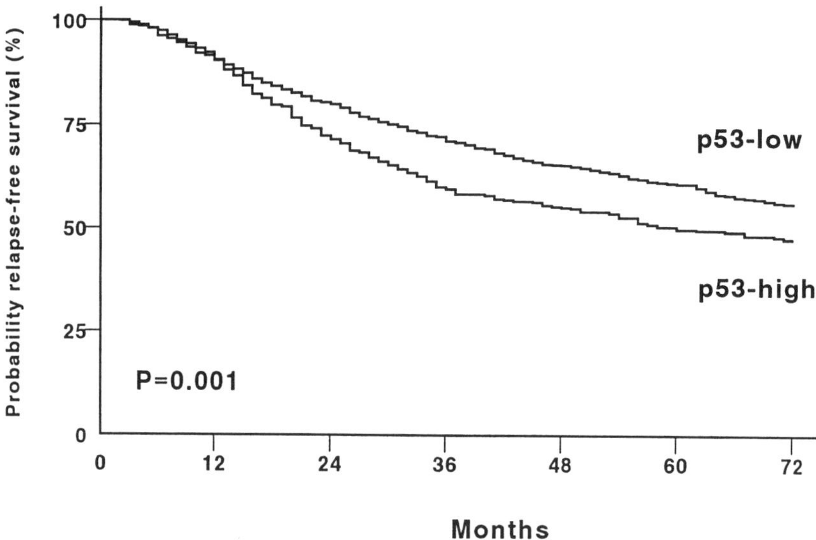

Fig. 3. Relapse-free survival as a function of p53 status in patients with primary breast cancer (cutoff value: 0.38 ng/mg protein, as explained in the text).

ing the rate of relapse. The relative hazard rate (RHR) with 95% confidence limits (CL) was 1.39 (1.19-1.63). This study supplements those of Thor et al. [27], Andersen et al. [28], or Elledge et al. [26], who also observed a relationship between immunohistochemically assessed p53 protein accumulation and shorter relapse-free survival, and confirms that of Borg et al. [21] who employed the same assay as we used in this study. Many reports, most of them based on p53 immunohistochemistry, suggest an association with well known indicators of high malignant potential such as high proliferation activity, high histological grade, elevated levels of tumour cells in S-phase and absence of ER and PgR, and with poor patient prognosis (review of 3000 breast cancer patients in [6,26]).

p53 and recurrent breast cancer

Endocrine and/or chemotherapy improves the prognosis for women with primary and advanced breast cancer. Extensive data suggest that p53 is a transcription factor that has "two faces" [29]: on the one hand p53 regulates cell cycle arrest and DNA repair, on the other hand it directs apoptosis (see Fig. 1). Lymphoid cells, for example, promptly undergo apoptosis after DNA damage. Apoptosis represents a mechanism whereby a variety of antitumour treatments result in cell death and cells with mutant p53 may be *resistant* to these forms of therapy. Conversely, cells with mutant p53, which are not likely to undergo apoptosis, may be more *sensitive* to certain (chemo)therapeutic drugs that produce DNA damage (such as doxorubicin, etoposide or cisplatin).

p53 levels and response to first-line tamoxifen therapy for recurrent disease

We have next evaluated the predictive value of p53 protein accumulation as measured by the LIA in cytosols prepared from primary breast tumours. One quarter of the patients studied above who underwent resection of the primary tumour between 1978-1991, developed recurrent disease and received tamoxifen (40 mg daily) as first-line hormonal therapy. After primary surgery only 19% of the patients received systemic adjuvant chemotherapy. The median age of these patients at the start of first-line tamoxifen therapy was 61 years. Patients were evaluated for response, and 49% responded to first-line tamoxifen therapy (complete or partial remission and stable disease over 6 months). As expected, postmenopausal patients (82%), patients with a longer disease-free interval (> 1 year; 68%), with a more favorable site of relapse or with ER-positive tumours (>10 fmol/mg protein; 86%) responded better to tamoxifen (Fig. 4). Based on p53 levels, the primary tumours were divided into 4 groups of equal size (quartiles). Patients with higher p53 levels in the primary tumour responded significantly worse to tamoxifen therapy (Fig. 5). Interestingly, those patients with lower ER values (< 75 fmol/mg protein) but high p53 levels in their primary tumours showed the poorest response (odds ratio: 0.37; 95% confidence limits: 0.19-0.71). Archer et al. [30], however, showed no significant relation between p53 expression assessed by immunohistochemistry, and response to endocrine treatment in a smaller series of patients with advanced disease,

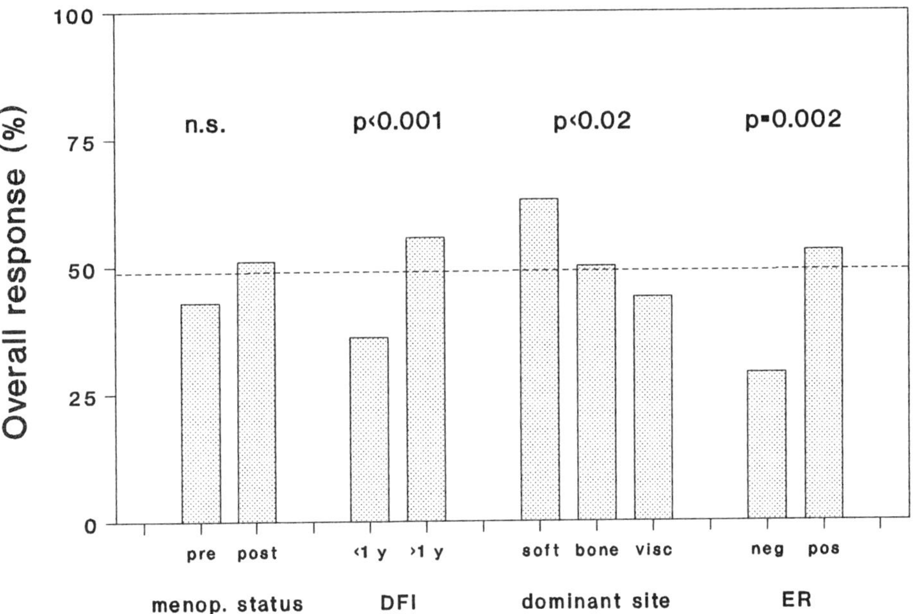

Fig. 4. Reponse to first-line tamoxifen therapy in the subset of patients with recurrent breast cancer. The dotted line represents the overall response rate of 49%.

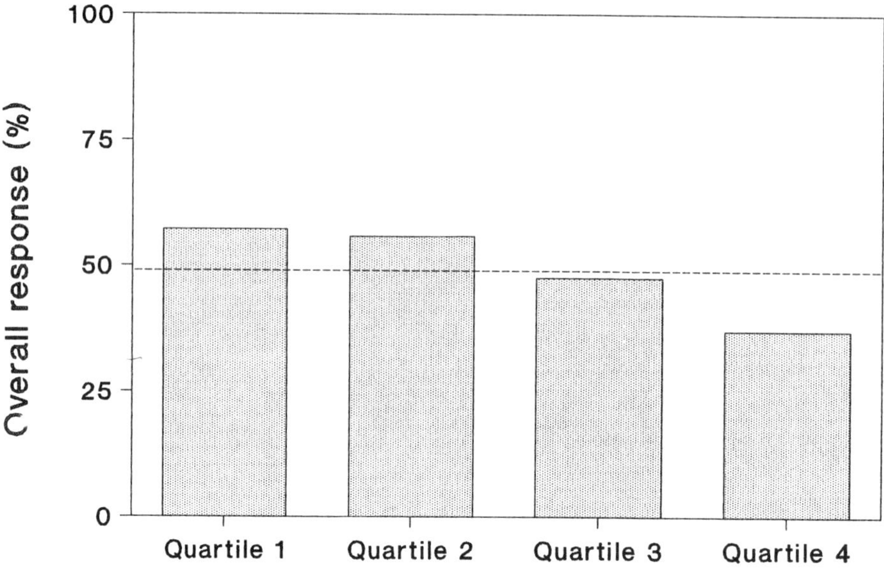

Fig. 5. Response to first-line tamoxifen therapy: p53 protein levels divided into four groups of equal size (quartiles). The dotted line represents the overall response rate of 49%.

whereas Horne et al. [31] showed that p53 overexpression was associated with a poor response to endocrine therapy. Tamoxifen therapy, along with radiotherapy, in the adjuvant setting seems to be of less value in patients with p53 gene mutations, as shown by Bergh et al. [32].

In conclusion, a high p53 protein level in the primary breast tumour is an independent predictor of poor response to first-line therapy with tamoxifen in recurrent breast cancers.

p53 levels and response to first-line polychemotherapy for recurrent disease

The predictive value of p53 protein accumulation with respect to the response to polychemotherapy was assessed in a small subset (6%) of patients. These patients underwent surgery between 1978 and 1991 and developed recurrent disease. The patients were given cyclophosphamide, methotrexate and 5-fluorouracil, CMF (70%), or cyclophosphamide, adriamycin and 5-fluorouracil, CAF (25%), or other forms of chemotherapy as first-line chemotherapy for recurrent disease. Seventy percent of the patients did not receive adjuvant treatment and 60% had ER-negative primary tumours. In 58% of the patients the dominant site of relapse was visceral. Of all patients studied in this subset, 47% responded to first-line chemotherapy (objective response and stable disease over 6 months). The tumours were ordered in four equal groups, based on the p53 levels of the primary tumours. Patients with the lowest and higher p53 levels in

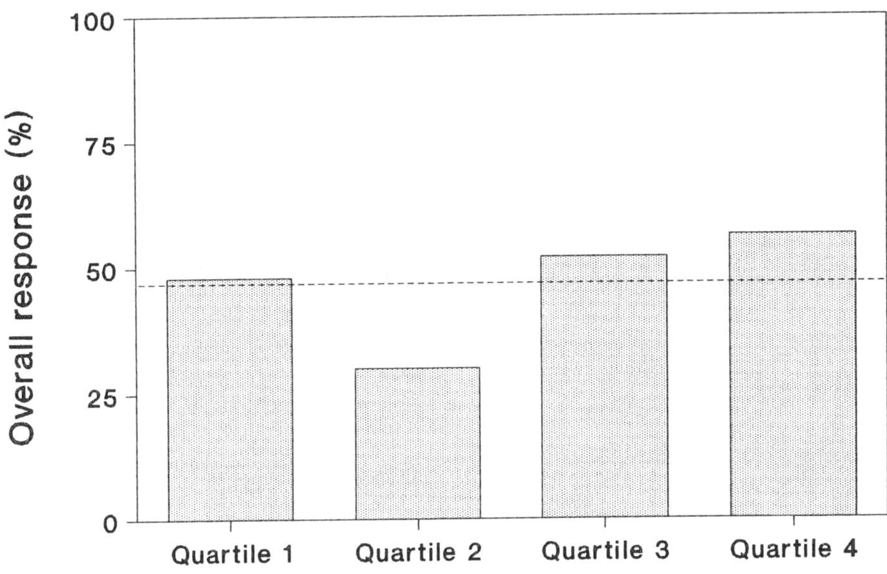

Fig. 6. Response to first-line polychemotherapy in a subset of patients: p53 protein levels divided into four groups of equal size (quartiles). The dotted line represents the overall response rate of 47%.

their primary tumours responded better to chemotherapy (Fig. 6), but this was not significant.

In conclusion, there is no relation between the p53 protein level in the primary breast tumour and response to first-line chemotherapy in recurrent breast cancer.

Comparison of LIA with SSCA/sequence analysis: a point of caution

The p53 gene has structural and functional similarities to the myc family of proto-oncogenes. Both p53 and myc gene alterations independently predict poor prognosis in breast cancer patients [34].

The LIA assay, which detects both wild-type and mutant p53 protein, is based on the principle that mutated p53 has a prolonged half-life and is thus accumulated in the cell. In a small subset of 151 primary breast tumour samples the LIA values were related to SSCA (exons 5-8) and subsequent sequence analysis. The median p53 level in 46 tumours with missense mutations, 4.2 ng/mg protein (range 0.0-176.0), was eight times higher than the level measured in 10 tumours with silent mutations, 0.5 ng/mg (range 0.0-11.9), or than the median level of 91 tumours without a p53 gene alteration, 0.4 ng/mg (range 0.0-70.8 ng/mg protein), but also than the level measured in 4 tumours with deletions/insertions, 0.6 ng/mg (range 0.0-13.0 ng/mg protein). Unfortunately these latter al-

62   E.M.J.J. Berns, J.A. Foekens and J.G.M. Klijn

32   Bergh J, Norberg T, Sjögren S, Lindgren A, Holmberg L. Complete sequencing of the p53 gene provides prognostic information in breast cancer patients, particularly in relation to adjuvant systemic therapy and radiotherapy. Nature Med 1995; 1: 1029-34
33   Harper JW, Adami GR, Wei N, Keyomarsi K, Elledge SJ. The p21 Cdk-interacting protein Cip1 is a potent inhibitor of G1 cycling-dependent kinases. Cell 1993; 75: 805-16
34   Berns EMJJ, Klijn JGM, Smid M et al. TP53 and myc gene alterations independently predict poor prognosis in breast cancer patients. Genes, Chromosomes & Cancer 1996; 16: 170-9

ESO Scientific Updates, Vol. 1
Prognostic and Predictive Value of p53
J.G.M. Klijn, editor

p53 Status: Impact on Breast Tumour Biology and Response to Therapy

Richard M. Elledge[1] and D. Craig Allred[2]

1   Division of Medical Oncology and Division of Radiation Oncology
2   Department of Pathology
    University of Texas Health Science Center, San Antonio, Texas, U.S.A.

Introduction

In the past, biomarkers associated with outcome have usually been lumped into a single defining category, labeled "prognostic factors", with little or no effort to distinguish between a factor's ability to assess biological aggressiveness versus response to therapy. The majority of prognostic factor studies combined or did not clearly distinguish between these two separate functions. As it has become apparent that systemic therapies for breast cancers are clearly, though modestly, effective and the number of therapeutic options have grown, it has become increasingly important to know whether an individual patient will respond to a specific therapy, so that the optimal therapy can be chosen for each patient. This discussion on p53 begins with specific definitions and clarifications of the terms prognostic and predictive factor.

A prognostic factor is indicative of the inherent biological aggressiveness of a tumour, reflecting the natural history of the disease after local therapy. It is, therefore, most accurately assessed in systemically untreated patients. An example of a prognostic factor is axillary nodal status. A predictive factor indicates the likelihood of a therapeutic response to a particular treatment. Study designs assessing predictive value are more complex because of additional variables involved. An example of a predictive factor for hormonal therapy is oestrogen receptor (ER). It is important to keep in mind that prognostic and predictive properties are not mutually exclusive and that a given factor can be both prognostic and predictive, as is the case with ER. Given these definitions, is p53 a prognostic factor, a predictive factor, or both?

Address for correspondence: R.M. Elledge, Division of Medical Oncology, University of Texas Health Science Center, 7703 Floyd Curl Drive, San Antonio, Texas 78284-7884, U.S.A. Tel.: +1-210-5674777, Fax: +1-210-5676687, e-mail: elledge@uthscsa.edu

Biological rationale supporting p53 as a prognostic factor

A starting point to answering this question is to examine whether there is a clear biological rationale for p53 in these roles. The p53 gene (and its protein) is by far the most heavily studied molecule in the human genome. Its functions are so diverse and widespread one wonders at times whether a single protein actually is involved in such a vast array of cellular functions. At the most basic level, p53 is a nuclear phosphoprotein that functions as a transcription factor [1,2]. It can bind to a p53 consensus element in a number of genes such as the human ribosomal gene cluster [3], muscle creatine kinase [4], mdm-2 [5], and WAF-1 [6], and in binding, it activates the transcription of these genes. It also inhibits the transcription of another set of genes containing TATA sequences in their promoter [7] by binding to elements of the basal transcription machinery [8]. Thus, p53 is a transcriptional modulator which can either turn on or off crucial genes. It also inhibits DNA replication [9,10] and is a checkpoint control molecule for progression from G1 to S-phase of the cell cycle [11]. By these general mechanisms, wild-type p53 slows proliferation. p53 is also involved in facilitating apoptosis [12], though p53-independent pathways for apoptosis also exist [13].

When p53 is inactivated either by mutation, loss, sequestration, or binding to other proteins, the cell may escape down the path of transformation. Cells with inactivated p53 generally have an increased proliferative rate [14], higher amounts of genomic instability [15], and lose their G1 to S checkpoint [16]. Under some conditions, loss of p53 function can result in resistance to apoptosis [17]. In breast cancer, inactivation of p53 is generally found in more advanced disease, with rates of inactivation between 0 and 15% for non-invasive breast cancers and between 20% and 50% for invasive breast cancers [18].

p53 and breast cancer prognosis

Because inactivation of p53 is more common in advanced breast cancer, results in increased proliferation and resistance to apoptosis, inactivation of p53 should be associated with a worse prognosis. There have been at least 50 studies in the published literature examining the association of p53 inactivation and prognosis in breast cancer. These studies are heterogeneous and in fact are not "pure" prognostic factor studies since many or most of them are based on mixed populations of systemically treated and untreated patients. Techniques for assessing inactivation of p53 also vary widely. The most common technique used is immunohistochemistry to assess accumulation of p53 protein; missense mutations frequently result in a prolonged protein half-life and protein accumulation. Fewer studies have used DNA-based techniques and an even smaller number have used RNA-based cDNA techniques. In these studies, inactivation of the p53 gene or protein, measured in various ways, is consistently associated with a number of other known poor prognostic factors, including oestrogen receptor (ER) negativity [19,20], progesterone receptor (PgR) negativity [21], high proliferative fraction [22], and poor nuclear/histological grade [23]. Interestingly, p53 status is generally not strongly associated with tumour size or nodal status. There is no clear or consistent difference in rates of p53 inactivation between node-positive and node-negative breast cancer [21]. Inactivation of p53 is also associated with a poor outcome as measured by disease-free survival or overall survival. In 33 studies totalling approximately 8,000 patients, inactivation of p53 was associated with a worse outcome. These findings are balanced against 17 publications involving 3,300 patients, which failed to demonstrate a significantly worse overall or disease-free survival. A number of these latter studies showed trends towards a worse outcome which did not reach statistical significance. It is interesting to note that the mean sample size in the positive studies was 240 while in the studies which did not show significance it was considerably smaller, approximately 190, suggesting that failure to show a significant difference may in part be due to insufficient statistical power.

Overall, one can conclude from the aggregate of these studies that inactivation of p53 is associated with a worse prognosis and increases the relative risk of relapse by approximately 1.3-1.5, i.e., 30-50%. This difference in risk of relapse between p53 inactivated and p53 wild-type or normal tumours is unfortunately not large enough to make p53 status alone clinically useful for making decisions about whether to use adjuvant systemic therapy. A significant portion of patients with p53 wild-type tumours still experience relapse, certainly above a threshhold of 10%, which is a consensus figure above which many oncologists would initiate systemic therapy.

Because many studies, including our own, contain a mixture of both treated and untreated patients, it is difficult to determine with certainty whether the generally worse outcome seen is due to a more aggressive tumour, resistance to systemic therapy or both. In order to more clearly test the hypothesis that p53 status is a prognostic factor, we surveyed our tumour bank and selected only patients who did not receive systemic therapy. There were 694 systemically untreated, node-positive and node-negative patients involved in this analysis [21,24]. Immunohistochemistry (IHC) status was assessed on frozen tumour specimens using a cocktail of antibodies 1801 and 240. Based on a prospective cutpoint analysis, a tumour was deemed positive if there was any detectable nuclear IHC staining. The results are seen in Figure 1. There was a highly significant difference in both disease-free (DFS) and overall survival (OS) between p53 IHC-positive patients (a non-functional phenotype) and p53 IHC-negative patients (normal function). When patients were separated into node-negative and node-positive groups, disease-free and overall survival patterns for both groups were the same, in that IHC-positive patients did significantly worse than IHC-negative patients (Fig. 1). In a multivariate analysis which included tumour size, nodal status, ER, PgR, and age, IHC positivity was independently associated with a worse outcome in these systemically untreated patients, p=0.008, DFS, p=0.056, OS. In summary, this large study based on untreated patients suggests that p53 inactivation is associated with a worse clinical outcome, though its prognostic significance is not powerful enough alone for it to be used in clinical decision making.

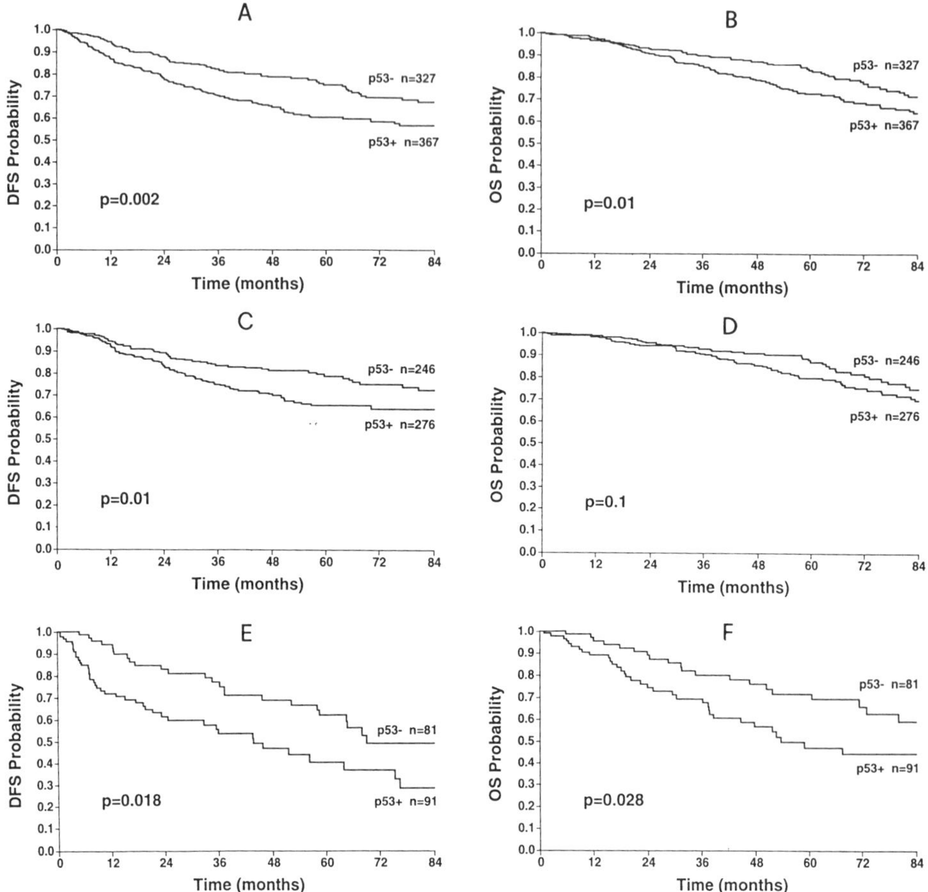

Fig 1. Disease-free and overall survival in systemically untreated breast cancer patients according to p53 status assessed by IHC. **A)** DFS, all patients. **B)** OS, all patients. **C)** DFS node-negative patients only. **D)** OS node-negative patients only. **E)** DFS node-positive patients. **F)** OS node-positive patients.

Oncological weather forecasting - issues of complexity and chaos

It is perhaps unrealistic and overly simplistic to expect that any individual biomarker alone will be prognostically powerful enough to be clinically useful. Cancer is a disease marked by multiple primary alterations in DNA, with each alteration leading to an ever widening cascade of secondary consequences and changes. There are then perhaps hundreds, or thousands, of changes in an individual cancer cell which contribute to its malignant behaviour. Additionally, within a tumour mass there is a large amount of heterogeneity between the billions of individual cells that form the mass, further increasing the complexity of the system. Underlying this complexity are probably a small number of "rules" or parameters that govern the initiation of the transformation process, though progression of this process is marked by randomness and chaos, making specific outcomes difficult to predict from an original set of conditions. In many respects, assessing clinical outcome using present biomarkers is analogous to planetary weather forecasting using barometric pressure and wind direction. The complexity and inherent disorder of both of these natural systems may necessitate the use of multiple integrated measurements to best and most accurately make predictions about future conditions. Perhaps hundreds of biological factors will have to be measured in order to achieve the goal of clinical utility.

Biological rationale supporting p53 as a predictive factor

Perhaps a more important question is whether p53 is a predictive factor in breast cancer. Before attempting to answer this, current and expanded models of mechanisms of action of systemic antineoplastic therapies will be briefly reviewed. It has long been thought that antineoplastic therapies, including chemotherapy and hormonal therapy, work through a variety of mechanisms, such as alkylation of DNA, interfering with nucleic acid synthesis, inhibition of key enzymes such as topoisomerases, general inhibition of protein synthesis, induction of DNA strand breakage, interference with tubulin metabolism, and blockage of hormone receptor interaction and growth factor expression. It is now becoming more apparent that these seemingly disparate mechanisms of action may share a distal final common pathway, apoptosis [25]. Anticancer therapies may ultimately generate signals that activate or open apoptotic metabolic pathways, for instance by damaging DNA or depriving cells of a crucial growth factor that inhibits apoptotic signals. Thus, a wide variety of commonly used agents in breast cancer may act simply by activating a distal apoptotic pathway. These agents include doxorubicin, 5-FU, paclitaxel, methotrexate, alkylating agents, and hormonal therapies such as oophorectomy, tamoxifen, and aromatase inhibitors. Additionally, while there are multiple known avenues of drug resistance, resistance may also come about through loss or inactivation of genes which stimulate apoptosis or activation or overexpression of apoptotic inhibitors such as bcl-2. Given the fact that p53 has been shown to be a crucial molecule modulating some apoptotic pathways and that drugs may exert their therapeutic effect through these apoptotic pathways, it can be hypothesized that alteration in p53 status could result in drug resistance. We therefore have conducted studies examining the relationship of p53 status to the two most common systemic therapies used in breast cancer today: tamoxifen and the combination of cyclophosphamide, methotrexate, and 5-FU (CMF).

p53 as a predictive factor in breast cancer - tamoxifen

The first therapy examined was tamoxifen. Since cells functionally deficient in p53 are resistant to apoptosis, and since oestrogen withdrawal [26], toremifene [27] and tamoxifen [28] can cause apoptosis *in vitro*, we hypothesized that inactivation of p53 could therefore result in a blockage of hormone-induced apoptosis and lead to clinical resistance. Preliminary data from our tumour bank supported this hypothesis, in that ER-positive, node-negative patients who received tamoxifen only as systemic therapy experienced a significantly improved disease-free survival only if their tumour had a functional p53 protein, as manifested by lack of protein detected by IHC accumulation, whereas patients whose tumours had positive IHC staining (inactivated p53) did not benefit from tamoxifen treatment (data not shown). This was a non-randomised, retrospective analysis, so in order to carry these observations further, *in vitro* experiments were done in which MCF-7 cells, which are wild-type for p53 and are tamoxifen sensitive, were transfected with a plasmid containing a cDNA of mutant 179 p53. Protein expression was assessed in a number of different clones, both by Western blotting and by immunohistochemistry. Response to tamoxifen was compared between parental cell lines, vector-only transfected control clones and mutant transfected clones in monolayer and soft agar conditions.

To briefly summarise the results (Fig. 2), these experiments failed to demonstrate that abrogation of p53 function through introduction of large amounts of mutant p53 protein results in tamoxifen resistance under either monolayer conditions or in soft agar (data not shown) [29].

Because *in vitro* experiments are subject to a variety of methodological artifacts, we then chose to test the hypothesis that p53 abrogation can result in tamoxifen resistance in human breast tumours. Paraffin blocks were retrospectively collected from patients who were entered prospectively onto a Southwest Oncology Group trial, 8228 [30]. In this trial, approximately 360 patients with ER-positive metastatic breast cancer who had measurable or evaluable disease received daily tamoxifen as initial metastatic therapy. The trial was begun in 1982 and completed accrual in 1987. Follow-up was at least 8 years. Tumour specimens were evaluated by immunohistochemistry for nuclear accumulation of p53 protein. p53 status was compared with tumour and patient characteristics, response, time to treatment failure, and survival [31]. In this study, antibody 1801 was used to evaluate accumulation of nuclear p53. Tumours were scored according to the proportion of tumour cells positively stained and if greater than 10% of cells stained positive, the tumour was deemed to be positive for inactivated p53. We first correlated p53 with tumour characteristics and found, consistent with published observations, that accumulation of p53 was statistically associated with low ER (less than 50 fmols/mg), p=0.002. p53 positivity was also strongly correlated with lower levels of bcl-2, p=0.004. Responses to tamoxifen of p53-positive vs. p53-negative tumours were virtually the same, with 58% of tumours responding that were IHC positive and 50% that were IHC negative, p=0.36. Time to treatment failure, perhaps a better

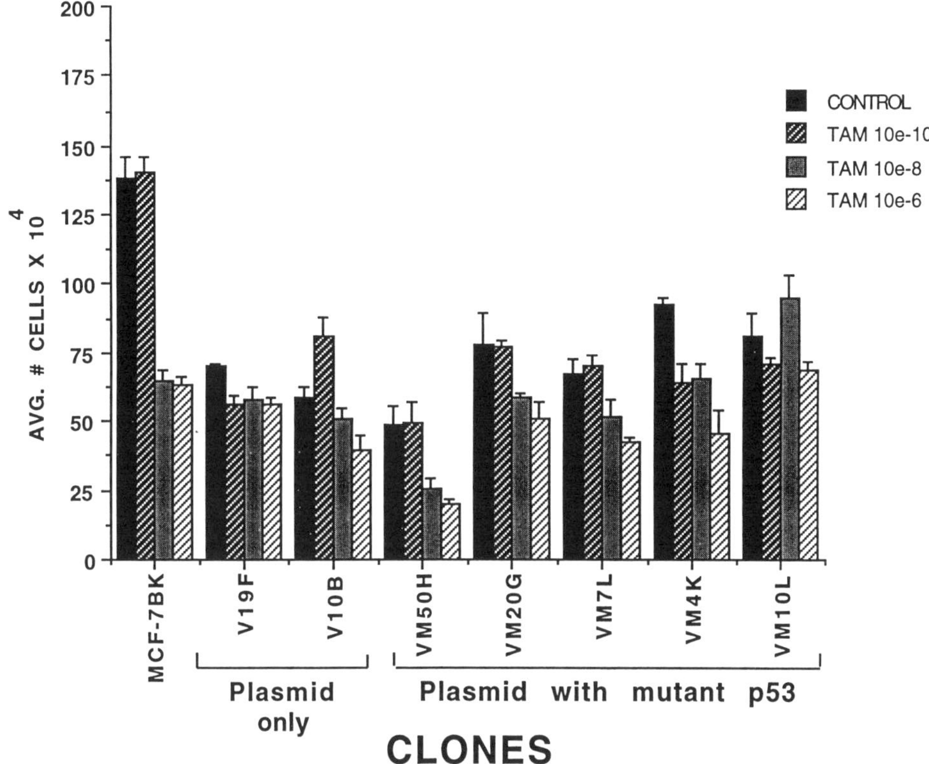

Fig. 2. Growth of clones and parental cell lines in various concentrations of 4-hydroxyta-moxifen (TAM). Cells (2 X 10^4) were plated and grown in MEM medium with 10% stripped FBS, 10^{-10} M estradiol, and the concentrations of 4-hydroxytamoxifen shown. Cells were grown for 6 days and counted at 50-75% confluency. All clones were grown in triplicate. Bars, SEM.

measurement of patient benefit from systemic therapy, was also examined. Time to treatment failure was not significantly longer in p53-negative patients, 8 months, than in p53-positive patients, 6 months (p=0.17). We also evaluated overall survival (Fig. 3). Patients with > 10% positively stained tumour cells had a significantly worse survival. Median survival was 20 months for patients who were IHC positive, but 36 months for those who were IHC negative. Five-year survival was 11% for those with a higher portion of positively stained cells versus 25% with fewer or no p53-altered cells. After adjusting for other potentially important variables, p53 remained an important factor in predicting survival, p=0.05.

From the above experiments and observations several conclusions can be drawn. First, *in vitro* inactivation of p53 does not result in resistance to tamox-ifen. In human breast tumours, p53 status as determined by IHC is not signifi-

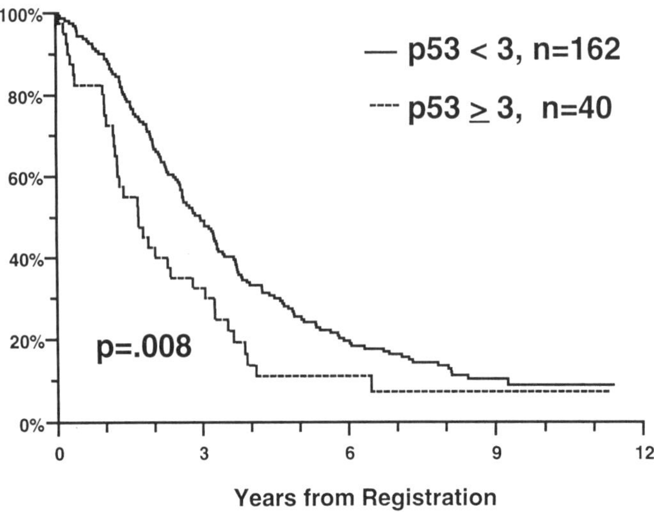

Fig. 3. Survival of patients according to IHC score. Patients with nuclear accumulation of p53 in greater than 10% of tumour cells (IHC score ≥ 3) had a worse survival.

cantly associated with response to tamoxifen although breast tumours with altered p53 protein are inherently more aggressive even after they have metastasised.

p53 as a predictive factor in breast cancer - CMF

We next turned our attention to looking at the predictive value of p53 status in relationship to cytotoxic therapy, i.e., CMF. It is known that restoration of p53 function and some p53 deficient or mutated cell lines results in apoptosis [32,33] and that cells with an intact p53 are more sensitive to DNA damaging agents *in vitro* and *in vivo* [34-37]. These observations suggest that p53 mutation might predict clinical resistance to chemotherapy. Indeed, one could hypothesize that in p53 wild-type cells, irreparable DNA damage caused by drugs results in apoptosis and this is manifested as a drug response (Fig. 4). Reparable damage in wild-type p53 cells would result in a G1 arrest, allowing time for repair of the damaged template. If DNA damage occurs in p53 mutated or inactivated cells there may be little if any growth arrest, no pause in G1, and decreased apoptosis, all of which would manifest clinically in resistance to therapy. To test this hypothesis we retrospectively collected paraffin block sections of tumours from patients treated on intergroup trial, INT 0011 [38]. In this trial, patients were required to be node-negative and treated with mastectomy. High-risk patients, i.e., those defined as being either ER-negative or having a tumour size greater than 3 cm, were randomised to receive CMFP or observation. Blocks

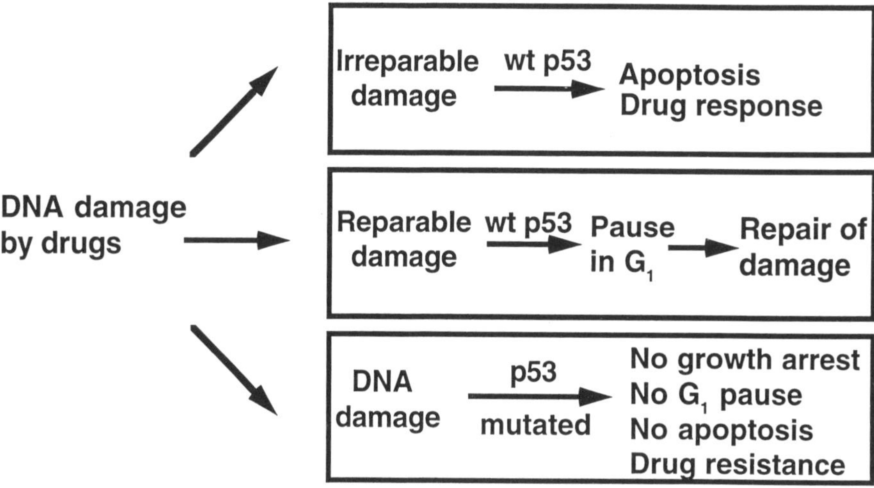

Fig. 4. Hypothesis explaining the mechanism of action of DNA damaging agents as a function of p53 status.

were available from 261 of these randomised patients and p53 status was evaluated by immunohistochemistry using antibody 1801. The median follow-up for this study was 8 years. Results of IHC staining were compared to time to treatment failure and survival, as seen in Figure 5 [39]. Examination of these unadjusted Kaplan-Meier plots suggests that the treatment effect was larger in the p53-negative group, indicating sensitivity. However, in a Cox regression model which analysed time to treatment failure and survival in relation to treatment, age, ER status, tumour size, nuclear and histological grade, S-phase and p53 status, there was no statistically significant interaction between p53 and treatment (p=0.16 for time to treatment failure and p=0.09 for survival). While there was a trend towards a larger treatment effect in p53-negative patients, the results were not statistically significant. Unfortunately, no clear conclusion emerges from this clinical experiment. Because of the modest effects of CMFP, the study may have been statistically underpowered to optimally address the questions of resistance to cytotoxic chemotherapy in relation to p53 status.

Explanations for the failure to demonstrate predictive value of p53 in breast cancer

Clinical data on p53 as a predictive factor to cytotoxic therapy is not consistent and unfortunately falls short of supporting the hypothesis that abrogation of p53 would result in resistance to cytotoxic chemotherapy. There are a number of possible explanations for this finding. First, because overall differences in treatment vs. no treatment are modest for present therapies, large numbers of

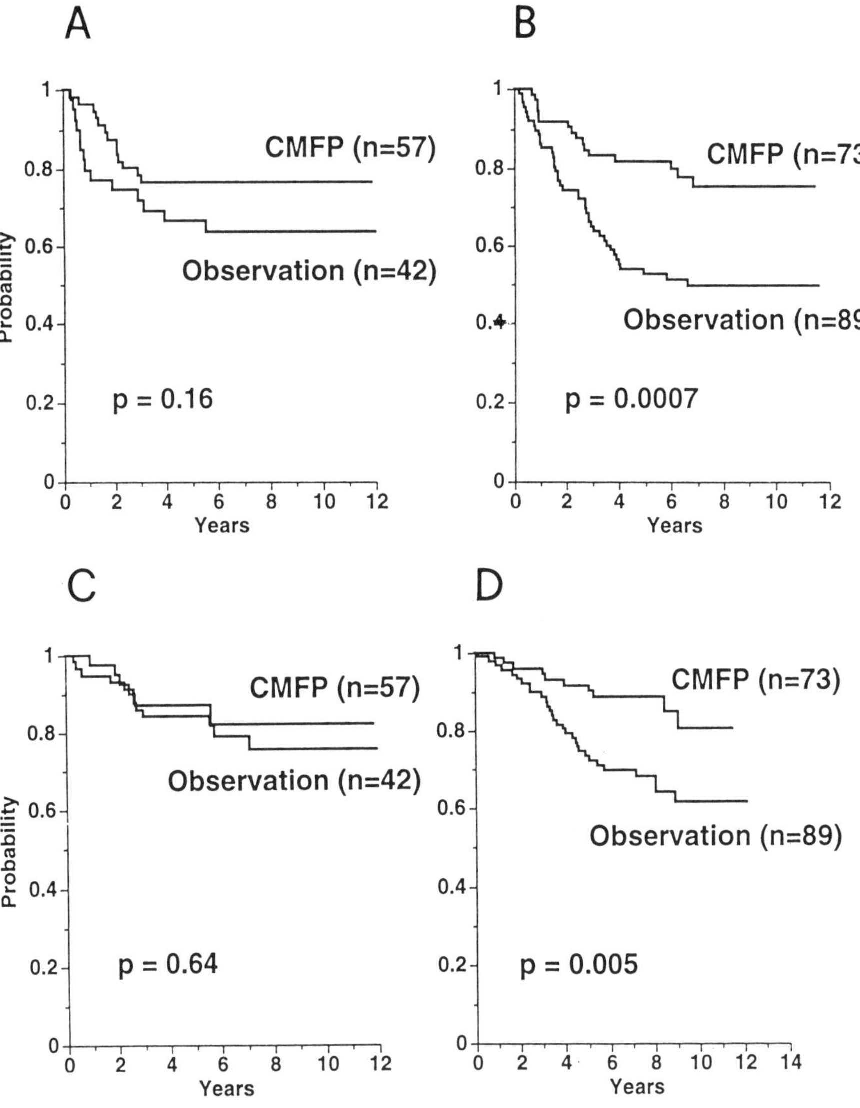

Fig. 5. Treatment effects for IHC p53-positive and IHC p53-negative patients. Patients are from the high-risk group who were randomly selected to be observed (obs) or to receive CMFP. **A)** Time to treatment failure for p53-positive patients. **B)** Time to treatment failure for p53-negative patients who were observed or who received CMFP. **C)** Overall survival for p53-positive patients who were observed or who received CMFP. **D)** Overall survival for p53-negative patients who were observed or who received CMFP. Although the graphical representations of the data suggest that patients with p53-negative tumours had a better response to therapy, there was no statistically significant interaction between CMFP treatment and p53 status as determined by IHC.

patients would be needed to have a statistical power large enough to detect this modest difference and, thus, studies may simply be too small to reliably detect an effect of such a small magnitude. Next, there is certainly evidence of multiple alternative apoptotic pathways that do not depend on p53 and apoptotic signals created by cytotoxic agents may flow down these alternate pathways. Also, the phenotypic, genotypic and cellular context in which apoptotic signals are received are important in determining whether these signals can be executed and what the final result may be. Thus, stimulation of a particular apoptotic pathway may produce different results, even in the same cell type, if the genetic changes or physiological environment against which these alterations occur are different. Present methods commonly used as surrogate markers of p53 function, namely protein accumulation and mutation detection, may be inaccurate at actually assessing function. Direct functional assays [40,41] or measurement of downstream components of the p53 pathways, such as p21, may be better indicators of p53 integrity. A final consideration is that *in vivo* and *in vitro* models in which resistance to cytotoxic chemotherapy have been observed with abrogation of p53 function may not be applicable to human breast tumours. Certainly, methodological artifacts can occur in transfection and transgenic models when genes are randomly integrated into the genome and are driven by non-native promoters. The biological systems created by these types of changes are artificial and prone to possible artifactual results.

Methodology and trial design for optimally evaluating the predictive value of p53

If results are not clear as to the predictive nature of p53, what is the way forward? Because ultimately the predictive value of p53 status must be assessed on large numbers of specimens derived from clinical trials, it is important that the method utilised is reproducible, accurate, and has a high throughput so that it can be performed on a large number of specimens. Efforts are now ongoing in this area using automated sequencing, direct functional assays [40,41], or high density oligonucleotide arrays on solid state supports [42] (DNA chip technology), the latter of which can be used to assess the downstream components of p53 and thus indirectly assess function. Another important aspect to be addressed is the trial design in which one seeks to assess the predictive value of p53. An adequate sample size is vital in breast cancer, a very heterogeneous disease where treatment effects are somewhat modest. The sample sizes should range in the hundreds when studying patient populations with metastatic or locally advanced disease and should be in the thousands when assessing the effect of p53 status in the adjuvant setting. Trials utilising smaller numbers of patients than this are prone to produce results that occur by chance alone. When designing the trial, if a cutpoint is to be used, that cutpoint should have a biological rationale and should always be defined prospectively. Researchers should avoid retrospective designations of cutpoints or searching for optimal cutpoints which, again, can lead to erroneous conclusions. Ideally, the population in which the predictive value of p53 is being assessed should be uniformly treated with a single agent so that if one has a "positive" result, one knows to which drug this result can be attributed. When patients are given multi-drug regimens it is impossible to sort this out. Perhaps the ideal trial design which gives the most reliable answer in the shortest amount of time is to select patients receiving initial systemic therapy for metastatic disease, define the trial prospectively and treat with a single agent. Other trial designs that are possible are neoadjuvant trials utilising core-needle biopsies (rather than fine-needle aspirates) and performing biopsies along a time course. Results of this type of trial are more immediately available because long follow-up is not needed and when multiple samples are obtained, one can gain a molecular, mechanistic insight from the observations. Studies done in the adjuvant setting are much more difficult because of the large numbers of patients needed and patients need to be randomised to at least two arms: one arm which receives treatment and one arm which receives no treatment or a randomisation which involves two arms where there is only a single treatment variable between each arm. In the adjuvant setting, these types of design are necessary to separate out the prognostic versus the predictive value of p53.

Conclusion

In summary, abrogation of p53 function results in a more aggressive tumour biology and a worse outcome for patients with breast cancer, regardless of stage. It is unclear whether p53 status provides additional information as to whether patients will respond to systemic therapy. More well-designed prospective clinical trials are needed along with rapid, accurate, and reproducible methods to assess p53 function. Up to now, the story of p53 has been an enlightening and exciting one and the promise for future developments remains bright.

References

1   Raycroft L, Wu H, Lozano G. Transcriptional activation by wild-type but not transforming mutants of the p53 anti-oncogene. Science 1990; 249: 1049-51
2   Farmer G, Bargonetti J, Zhu H, Friedman P, Prywes R, Prives C. Wild-type p53 activates transcription in vitro. Nature 1992; 358: 83-6
3   Kern S, Kinzler K, Bruskin A et al. Identification of p53 as a sequence-specific DNA-binding protein. Science 1991; 252: 1708-11
4   Zambetti G, Bargonetti J, Walker K, Prives C, Levine A. Wild-type p53 mediates positive regulation of gene expression through a specific DNA sequence element. Genes & Development 1992; 6: 1143-52
5   Wu X, Bayle J, Olson D, Levine A. The p53-mdm-2 autoregulatory feedback loop. Genes & Development 1993; 7: 1126-32
6   El-Deiry W, Tokino T, Velculescu V et al. WAF1, a potential mediator of p53 tumor suppression. Cell 1993; 75: 817-25

7   Mack D, Vartikar J, Pipas J, Laimins L. Specific repression of TATA-mediated but not initiator-mediated transcription by wild-type p53. Nature 1993; 363: 281-3

8   Thut C, Chen J, Klemm R, Tjian R. p53 transcription activation mediated by coactivator $TAF_{II}40$ and $TAF_{II}60$. Science 1995; 267: 100-4

9   Cox L, Hupp T, Midgley C, Lane D. A direct effect of activated human p53 on nuclear DNA replication. EMBO J 1995; 14: 2099-105

10   Dutta A, Ruppert J, Aster J, Winchester E. Inhibition of DNA replication factor RPA by p53. Nature 1993; 365: 79-82

11   Lin D, Shields M, Ullrich S, Appella E, Mercer W. Growth arrest induced by wild-type p53 protein blocks cells prior to or near the restriction point in late G1 phase. Proc Natl Acad Sci 1992; 89: 9210-4

12   Yonish-Rouach E, Resnitzky D, Lotem J, Sachs L, Kimchi A, Oren M. Wild-type p53 induces apoptosis of myeloid leukaemic cells that is inhibited by interleukin-6. Nature 1991; 352: 345-7

13   Clarke A, Purdie C, Harrison D, Morris R, Bird C, Hooper M, Wyllie A. Thymocyte apoptosis inducted by p53-dependent and independent pathways. Nature 1993; 362: 849-52

14   Runnebaum I, Yee J-K, Kieback D, Sukumar S, Friedmann T. Wild-type p53 suppresses the malignant phenotype in breast cancer cells containing mutant p53 alleles. Anticancer Res 1994; 14: 1137-44

15   Livingstone L, White A, Sprouse J, Livanos E, Jacks T, Tisty T. Altered cell cycle arrest and gene amplification potential accompany loss of wild-type p53. Cell 1992; 70: 923-35

16   Mercer W, Shields M, Amin M et al. Negative growth regulation in a glioblastoma tumor cell line that conditionally expresses human wild-type p53. Proc Natl Acad Sci 1990; 87: 6166-70

17   Symonds H, Krall L, Remington L et al. p53-dependent apoptosis suppresses tumor growth and progression in vivo. Cell 1994; 78: 703-11

18   Davidoff A, Kerns B, Inglehard J, Marks J. Maintenance of p53 alterations throughout breast cancer progression. Cancer Res 1991; 51: 2605-10

19   Isola J, Visakorpi T, Holli K, Kallioniemi O-P. Association of overexpression of tumor suppressor protein p53 with rapid cell proliferation and poor prognosis in node-negative breast cancer patients. J Natl Cancer Inst 1992; 84: 1109-14

20   Thorlacius S, Børresen A-L, Eyfjörd J. Somatic p53 mutations in human breast carcinomas in an Icelandic population: a prognostic factor. Cancer Res 1993; 53: 1637-41

21   MacGrogan G, Bonichon F, Mascarel I et al. Prognostic value of p53 in breast invasive ductal carcinoma: an immunohistochemical study on 942 cases. Br Cancer Res Treat 1995; 36: 71-81

22   Allred D, Clark G, Elledge R et al. Association of p53 protein expression with tumor cell proliferation rate and clinical outcome in node-negative breast cancer. J Natl Cancer Inst 1993; 85: 200-6

23   Thor A, Moore D, Edgerton S et al. Accumulation of p53 tumor suppressor gene protein: An independent marker of prognosis in breast cancers. J Natl Cancer Inst 1992; 84: 845-55

24   Allred D, Clark G, Fuqua S et al. Overexpression of p53 in node-positive breast cancer. Br Cancer Research Treat 1993; 27: 131

25   Hickman J. Apoptosis induced by anticancer drugs. Cancer and Metastasis Review 1992; 11: 121-39

26   Kyprianou N, English H, Davidson N, Isaacs J. Programmed cell death during regression of the MCF-7 human breast cancer following estrogen ablation. Cancer Res 1991; 51: 162-6

27   Wärri A, Huovinen R, Laine A, Martikainen P, Härkönen P. Apoptosis in toremifene-induced growth inhibition of human breast cancer cells in vivo and in vitro. J Natl Cancer Inst 1993; 85: 1412-8

28   Perry R, Kang Y, Greaves B. Effects of tamoxifen on growth and apoptosis of estrogen-dependent and -independent human breast cancer cells. Ann Surg Oncol 1995; 2(3): 238-45
29   Elledge R, Lock-Lim S, Allred D, Hilsenbeck S, Cordner L. p53 mutation and tamoxifen resistance in breast cancer. Clin Cancer Res 1995; 1: 1203-8
30   Ravdin P, Green S, Door T et al. Prognostic significance of progesterone receptor levels in estrogen receptor-positive patients with metastatic breast cancer treated with tamoxifen: results of a prospective Southwest Oncology Group study. J Clin Oncol 1992; 10(8): 1284-91
31   Elledge R, Green S, Howes L et al. bcl-2, p53, and response to tamoxifen in ER-positive metastatic breast cancer: A Southwest Oncology Group study. J Clin Oncol 1997; 15 (5): 1916-22
32   Shaw P, Bovey R, Tardy S, Sahli R, Sordat B, Costa J. Induction of apoptosis by wild-type p53 in a human colon tumor-derived cell line. Proc Natl Acad Sci 1992; 89: 4495-9
33   Fujiwara T, Grimm E, Mukhopadhyay T, Cai D, Owen-Schaub L, Roth J. A retroviral wild-type p53 expression vector penetrates human lung cancer spheroids and inhibits growth by inducing apoptosis. Cancer Res 1993; 53: 4129-33
34   Fujiwara T, Grimm E, Mukhopadhyay T, Owen-Schaub L, Roth J. Induction of chemo-sensitivity in human lung cancer cells in vivo by adenovirus-mediated transfer of the wild-type p53 gene. Cancer Res 1994; 54: 2287-91
35   Lotern J, Sachs L. Hematopoietic cells from mice deficient in wild-type p53 are more resistant to induction of apoptosis by some agents. Blood 1993; 82(4): 1092-6
36   Lowe S, Ruley H, Jacks T, Housman D. p53-dependent apoptosis modulates the cyto-toxicity of anticancer agents. Cell 1993; 74: 957-67
37   Lowe S, Bodis S, McClatchey A et al. p53 status and the efficacy of cancer therapy in vivo. Science 1994; 266: 807-10
38   Mansour E, Gray R, Shatila A et al. Efficacy of adjuvant chemotherapy in high risk node-negative breast cancer. An intergroup study. N Engl J Med 1989; 320: 485-90
39   Elledge R, Gray R, Mansour E, Yu Y et al. Accumulation of p53 protein as a possible predictor of response to adjuvant combination chemotherapy with cyclophosphamide, methotrexate, fluorouracil, and prednisone for breast cancer. J Natl Cancer Inst 1995; 87(16): 1254-56
40   Frebour T, Barbier N, Kassel J, Ng Y-S, Romero P, Friend S. A functional screen for germ line p53 mutations based on transcriptional activation. Cancer Res 1992; 52: 6976-8
41   Friend S, Iggo R, Ishioka C, Fitzgerald M, Hoover I, O'Neill E, Frebourg T. Overcoming complexities in genetic screening for cancer susceptibility. Cold Spring Harbor Symposia on Quantitative Biology, Volume LIX, 1994; 673-6
42   Goffeau A. Molecular fish on chips. Nature 1997; 385: 202-3

ESO Scientific Updates, Vol. 1
Prognostic and Predictive Value of p53
J.G.M. Klijn, editor
© 1997 Elsevier Science B.V. All rights reserved

The Prognostic Significance and Interactions of p53 in Human Cancer

J.J. Anderson[1], J. Lunec[2], I. Sigalas[2], S.R. Al Tamimi[1], B. Angus[1], G.M. Horne[1] and C.H.W. Horne[1]

1   Department of Pathology, Unitersity of Newcastle-upon-Tyne
2   Cancer Research Unit, University of Newcastle-upon-Tyne, United Kingdom

The role of p53 in cell replication

The p53 gene resides within chromosome 17 at position 17p13.1. It is composed of 11 exons (10 coding) encompassing a region of DNA between 16-20kb. The protein product encoded is a highly phylogenetically conserved 53kDa nuclear phosphoprotein which binds to DNA in a sequence-specific manner and acts as a transcription factor intimately involved in regulation of proteins associated with the control of cell proliferation and apoptosis. It has been shown to express features characteristic of a tumour suppressor gene product and frequent primary mutations have been recorded in a variety of human cancers while germ-line mutations have been shown to be associated with predisposition to tumour development.

The active wild-type p53 tetramer has been proposed to act as a molecular switch which can define the fate of the proliferating cell by monitoring and ensuring the "integrity of the genome" as replication progresses through the G1-S phase transition [1]. The array of mechanisms through which the p53 protein expresses its activity have yet to be completely defined. However, a great deal of work has delineated the structure of the p53 molecule. It may be divided into three distinct regions: i) an acidic proline-rich amino-terminal region incorporating phosphorylation sites (targets of a DNA-dependent protein kinase) as well as regulatory protein binding sites involved in determining the transactivational ability of the molecule; ii) a central region involved in the formation of interactions with DNA, and iii) a carboxy-terminal region associated with nuclear localisation, multimer formation and "recognition" of DNA damage in the form of single stranded breaks [2].

Address for correspondence: J.J. Anderson, Department of Pathology, University of Newcastle-upon-Tyne, Newcastle-upon-Tyne NE1 4HH, United Kingdom.
Tel.: +44-191-2226000, ext. 8792, Fax: +44-191-2228100, e-mail: j.j.anderson@ncl.ac.uk

The function of p53 as a transcriptional regulator has received considerable attention. It is known to bind via its central conserved region (amino acids 100-300) to specific consensus DNA sequences represented in regulatory elements of target genes [3]. Activation of transcription is thought to involve interaction of the NH2-terminal region of p53 with TATA box binding protein-associated factors including TAF^{II}40 and TAF^{II}60 [4]. Among the products currently recognised as being subject to p53 transcriptional control are the cdk/PCNA inhibitor p21 [5], the IGF-BFP3 [6], GADD45 [7], bax [8] (positive regulation) and bcl-2 (negative regulation) [9, 10] genes as well as the mdm-2 "oncogene" [11]. The latter of these in its primary protein form is thought to act as an autocrine regulator of p53 activity, binding to a conserved site (amino acids 18-23) (block 1) within the acidic amino-terminal portion of the p53 molecule [12,13]. p53 protein synthesis and stabilisation is induced in response to DNA damage and other cellular stressors, and results in the transactivation of IGF-BF3 as well as p21, which suppresses the activity of cdk4-cyclin D and cdk2-cyclin E complexes in G1, as well as cdk2-cyclin A complexes in S/G2 phase, effectively inducing transient halts in cell replication (Fig. 1). These pauses are believed to prevent replication on a damaged DNA template and allow DNA repair mechanisms the opportunity to act and amend any damage. p53 itself may form part of the complexes involved in the processes of replication and repair. Inadequate repair and persistence of p53 induction then may lead either directly or indirectly to up-regulation of bax-1 and down-regulation of bcl-2, which may augment formation of bax-1 homodimers, and participate in the ini-

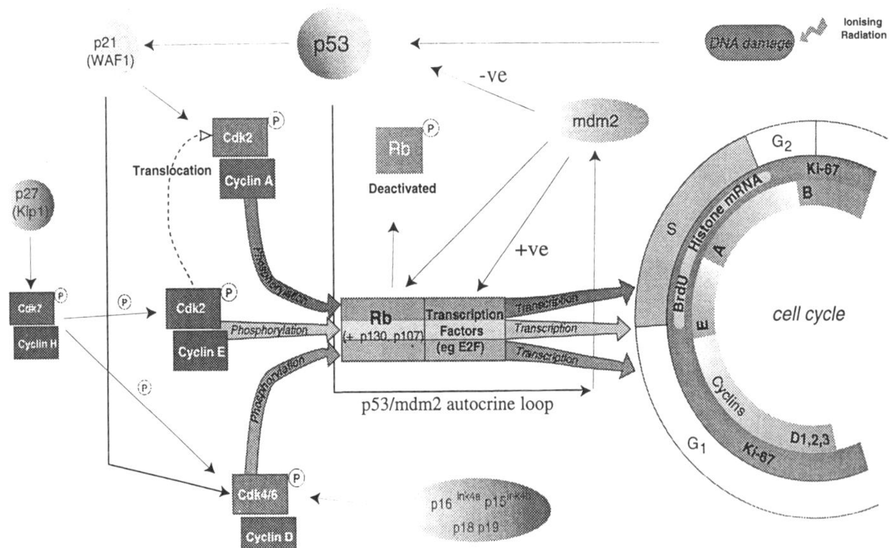

Fig. 1. p53 and mdm-2 control circuits operating to regulate the proliferation of the cell in response to genotoxic assault.

tiation of apoptosis, leading to the induction of the ICE-like proteases, chromatin condensation and ultimately to cell death. In addition, p53-mediated induction of p21 may also play a role in the induction of the apoptotic cascade [14]. These p53-dependent processes together help assure the elimination of the aberrant cell.

It is clear that defects in the structure and function of p53, or of p53 regulators, could deregulate the above control processes and could result in loss of transcriptional function, cell cycle checkpoint control and failure to undergo apoptosis. The net result would be further deterioration of genomic stability, deregulated cell growth and propagation of the aberrant phenotype.

The significance of p53 alterations

The sequence of p53 is strictly preserved, particularly within sequences encoding regions which determine those principal structural motifs (blocks II-V) which are critical for the maintenance of normal function. Mutations in the p53 gene, altering the structure and function of the encoded protein, have been described in up to 50% of human tumours including sarcomas, leukaemias, colonic, lung, oesophageal, bladder and breast carcinomas [15]. This is consistent with the central regulatory role of p53 encompassing pathways in the initiation and development of the process of oncogenesis. The observation that p53 null mice develop normally, but show an increased predisposition to cancer highlights the importance of additional molecular events in the induction of oncogenesis. The importance of such events in man is supported by the results of studies of patients with Li-Fraumeni syndrome, who have been found to possess heterozygous germ-line p53 mutations and also exhibit increased susceptibility to cancers.

Many studies have revealed that identifying functionally impaired forms of p53 within early cancer lesions may provide a means of predicting subsequent tumour behaviour and determining patient prognosis. Such information may potentially assist in directing patient treatment. Preliminary research has also indicated that assessment of tumour p53 conformation may possibly help in predicting the efficacy of response to anticancer therapy [16,17]. Furthermore, modulation of the effects of dysfunction through vectored gene therapy and competition with specific inhibitors could also provide novel opportunities for improved patient management and tumour-specific therapies. It is therefore essential that p53 structure and function can be accurately and rapidly assessed within a particular tumour. It is equally important that p53 is not thought of in isolation but in the wider context of the molecules through which it exerts its effects, as well as in the context of those regulators which impact upon it.

Immunohistochemical analysis of p53 protein expression

Several methods have been applied to assess p53 status in neoplastic tissues. Mutations have been shown to give rise to conformational variations which modify both the structure and physical characteristics of the molecule, the net functional results being both failure to bind to DNA and transactivational interference [4]. Physically, wild-type p53 has only a short half-life in the normal cell. Missense mutations in even a single allele of p53 can lead to the formation of protein complexes which may be inactive and display distinct physical characteristics. Such dysfunctional complexes are often dimers composed of an altered p53 molecule, being the product of a mutant allele, bound to and effectively inactivating a normal p53 molecule encoded by the remaining wild-type allele. These molecules display a protracted half-life which effects intranuclear accumulation of the disparate protein which may be detected using conventional immunohistochemical techniques. A variety of different polyclonal and monoclonal antibodies have been developed which primarily recognise dominant epitopes which appear on exposed surfaces of the amino and carboxy-terminal regions of the p53 molecule (Fig. 2). A number of these have been applied in immunohistochemistry to assess p53 status in sections of tumour tissue.

Breast cancer is the third most common cancer in the world today and by far the most common in women, with over half a million new cases arising annually [18]. As such it is a primary cause of mortality and improvements in the understanding of the pathogenesis as well as in management and treatment of the disease are the constant objectives of ongoing research.

Applying immunohistochemistry (IHC) to study nuclear p53 protein accumulation as a marker of p53 abnormality in breast cancers has demonstrated alterations in as many as 53.5% of tumours [19-24]. However, the selection of anti-

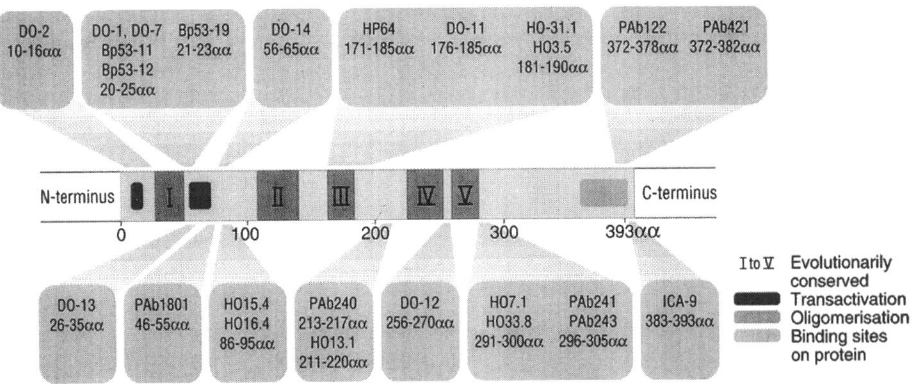

Fig. 2. Map of the human p53 molecule indicating the epitopes recognised by a variety of monoclonal antibodies which have been used to study p53 and their relationship to the positions of a number of the major functional elements of the molecule. (Reproduced with the consent of Novacastra Laboratories).

bodies applied in such studies can exert a strong influence upon the estimation of the frequency of occurrence of abnormalities as well as the conclusions drawn as to the prognostic significance of the observations. A number of comparative studies have examined the effect of applying different antibodies in parallel to assess the prognostic significance of p53 alterations [17,25,26]. In our laboratories we have compared antibodies PAb1801 (epitope: aa 46-55), DO7 (epitope: aa 20-25), p53-BP12 (epitope: aa 20-25) and polyclonal antibody CM1 [17]. In a series of 245 primary breast cancers nuclear accumulation of p53 could be detected using each of these antibodies when applying high temperature antigen unmasking techniques. However, a degree of discordance was apparent. p53-specific nuclear immunostaining was found to vary from 37.6% (CM1) to 46.8% (PAb1801). In addition, only data assembled from the assessment of p53 immunostaining which was made using PAb1801 indicated that nuclear accumulation of p53 protein was significantly related to reduced long-term patient survival (p=0.0171) (Fig. 3). Interestingly, this relationship was found to reside predominantly within the subgroup of patients whose lymph nodes did not

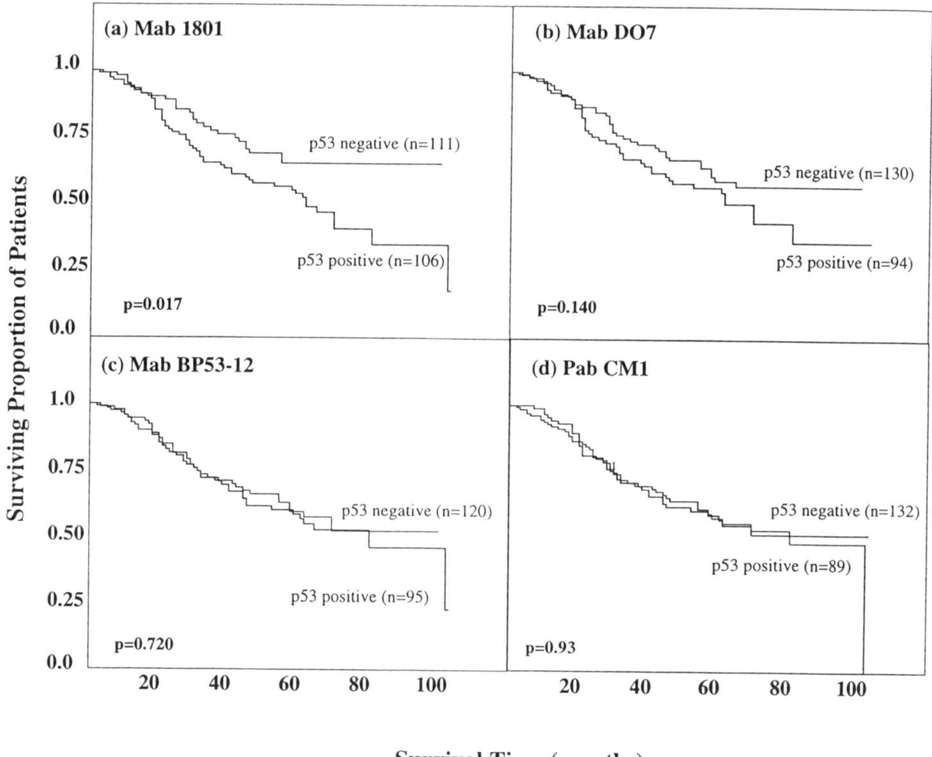

Fig. 3. Illustration of the effect which the choice of monoclonal antibody applied to detect nuclear accumulation of p53 in IHC may have upon the apparent significance of the marker as an indicator of long-term patient survival. (Fig. 3a reproduced from [17])

show any evidence of metastases (p=0.030), although a similar general trend was also observed among node-positive patients (p=0.169). In contrast to the variation observed with respect to patient survival, all four antibodies indicated that p53 nuclear immunostaining was associated strongly with high tumour grade. In addition, preliminary findings suggested an inverse relationship between nuclear p53 immunostaining and response to endocrine therapy [17].

The current considerable volume of data which has been derived from survival analyses based upon study of nuclear p53 accumulation as defined by IHC, has been recently reviewed and failed to categorically support its value as an independent indicator of reduced patient survival, although tumours collected from more than 9800 patients were studied [24]. However, strong correlations have been repeatedly reported between tumour p53 IHC positivity and established conventional markers of poor prognosis such as tumour grade and mitotic index, as well as more recently adopted IHC markers such as hormone receptor negativity and increased expression of c-erbB-2. In addition, associations have also been described with tumour aggressiveness and increased tendency to disease relapse, which in turn is found to concur with a general increase in the relative proportion of IHC p53-positive cells within the reccurring tumour [19,27,28]. In interpreting the results it must be remembered that in these studies not only do the antibodies used to detect nuclear p53 accumulation vary, but the methodologies employed in both IHC detection (indirect antibody, SAB, PAP etc.) and antigen retrieval, often applied to formalin-fixed tissues, may also be the subjects of considerable variation. Thus, standardisation to an optimal detection regime, which must always be influenced by the vagaries of the variable effects of non-uniform tissue fixation, is likely not to have been universally applied. The sum of currently available data has been taken to suggest that tumour nuclear p53 IHC positivity may be viewed as a likely indicator of poor patient prognosis/survival, perhaps of greatest value in predicting short-term (<60 months) prognosis but less reliable over longer periods (>100 months). However, it does not fulfil the criteria for a decisive-directive marker which would allow confident prediction of patient management, and its routine assessment has not been supported in the "Clinical Practice Guidelines for the Use of Tumour Markers in Breast Cancer" adopted and presented by the American Society of Clinical Oncology in October 1996 [27].

Molecular analysis of p53 gene abnormalities

Studies of the significance of abnormalities of p53 protein function and accumulation have been paralleled by a host of investigations which have sought to determine the frequency and nature of the genetic changes occurring within the p53 gene. A variety of molecular techniques have been applied to identify p53 gene alterations in breast and other cancers. These have included PCR amplification and direct dideoxygenic sequencing, single strand conformation polymorphism (SSCP) [28] and constant denaturant gradient gel electrophoresis (CDGE) [29]. Together these methods have described the occurrence of p53 mutations in

12% to 46% of invasive breast carcinomas [29], while loss of heterozygosity studies have reported changes occurring at the p53 locus in up to 64% of breast cancers [30]. In distinct geographical populations the incidence of p53 alterations may be even higher as recent data from Northern Japan has indicated that p53 alterations were detectable in 81% of tumours examined [31]. Missense mutations have been found to map predominantly within the DNA binding domain of p53, encompassing exons 5 to 8. As a result several assessments of the occurrence of p53 mutations have centred solely upon these regions (blocks II-V). However, research has shown that in breast as well as other tumours, mutations do occur outside this region (approximately 22%) and that the nature of these mutations may be different to those found within it [32]. It has been reported that few missense mutations and microdeletions occur outside this region, whereas frameshift mutations appear to occur more frequently in exons 2-4 and 9-11. These observations should be borne in mind when comparing the results of different studies which have effectively compared mutation rates in differing portions of the molecule, thereby presenting an incomplete picture and reduced estimate of p53 alteration. In addition, mutations within these less frequently studied areas, i.e., exons 2-4 and 9-11, may also exert major effects upon p53 expression and function given the nature of the frameshift mutations which predominate. Even those mutations occurring downstream of the DNA binding site are potentially important as major p53 nuclear localisation signal I (NLS-I) (aa 316-322) as well as minor NLS II and III map within exons 9 and 11, respectively, while the oligomerisation domain also resides within the C-terminal portion of the molecule.

In general, those studies which have centred in the main upon identification of missense mutations within the conserved DNA binding portion of the molecule have, in line with IHC studies, suggested that detection of p53 mutation may provide prognostically significant information [33-35], particularly among the node-negative patient group. In addition, these findings have reinforced the opinion that identification of p53 alterations may also be associated with rapid disease relapse and reduced short-term survival. Furthermore, associations have also been confirmed between genetic alterations in p53 and a variety of histo- and clinicopathological variables which have been reported as being associated which poor clinical outcome. These include hormone receptor (ER and PgR) negativity, high S-phase fraction (mitotic figure counts, Ki67 and cyclin A expression) and c-erbB-2 overexpression as well as high tumour grade [33,36,37]. However, some studies have failed to support a number of these associations [38]. Estimation of p53 mutations in populations of different racial origin has also suggested that the relevant prognostic significance of p53 alterations may vary with respect to the patients' ethnic origin [39].

Among those studies which have searched for mutations throughout exons 2-11, the prognostic significance of null mutations encoding truncated proteins has been found to be equally strongly associated with reduced clinical outcome as missense mutations which predominate between exons 5-9 and encode dysfunctional products [32,40].

Comparison of IHC and molecular analysis of p53 alterations

Immunohistochemical detection of nuclear p53 accumulation, in spite of all the problems of variabilitiy of detection systems and retrieval systems, has proved a valuable simple means of detecting p53 aberration but by its very nature it is unable to detect all the different aberrant forms of p53 which may arise. Study of the occurrence and nature of genetic alterations within the p53 gene has shown that agreement between identification of mutation and IHC detection of accumulation of p53 is incomplete. Mutations resulting in expression of a truncated protein, could fail to present epitopes which would be recognised by single monoclonal antibody probes. Other mutations, including homozygous deletions, could result in complete failure to produce a product. In addition, missense mutations could produce more subtle changes which could again affect epitope structure and recognition or even amenability to specific antigen retrieval. In each instance, IHC could fail to demonstrate nuclear accumulation of p53. Alterations could also result in loss of the ability of p53 to locate within the nucleus, where it must reside in order to exert its activity as a transactivational regulator. Indeed, one study has suggested that cytoplasmic IHC staining with p53-specific antibody has some prognostic value [41]. Conversely, mutations in p53 may arise which may alter its physiological function while not unduly prolonging its half-life, with the result that intranuclear accumulation of p53 may not be evident. Reports have described the occurrence of several of the above scenarios. The monoclonal antibody D07 has been reported to have failed to detect nuclear accumulation of p53 in tumours found to possess defined mutations, including single base pair insertions and deletions, which resulted in frameshift and creation of a new stop codon, respectively [28]. However, both appeared IHC positive when a second antibody, PAb1801, was applied as the detector. Conversely, reports have described tumours in which nuclear accumulation of p53 was evident but which were found to possess no detectable mutations. Such behaviour has been described in a variety of tumours in addition to breast, including colorectal, endometrial and gastric tumours [42]. This clearly raises the question of whether the accumulated wild-type p53 is functional and has led to the analysis of downstream mediators of p53 function to complement information on p53 status. In general, concordance of IHC and estimation of p53 gene alterations has been reported to vary between 68% and 79%, being highest in breast tumours.

p53 interactions: their prognostic significance

The activity of p53 may be modulated by a number of factors in addition to function modifying gene mutations. It has long been established that p53 may complex with and be inactivated by a number of "transforming" proteins encoded by oncogenic viruses, including the T antigen of SV40, the E6 protein of human papillomaviruses 16 and 18, and the E1B protein of adenovirus. The result of complex formation with these products is removal of functional p53 protein either as a direct result of complex formation, or by increasing ubiquitin-dependent breakdown. Recently, p53 has also been shown to form a complex with and be inactivated by the product of the human homologue of the mdm-2 gene [43,44]. The full-length product of this gene has been found to be a protein which has an apparent Mr, in PAGE, of 90-92K, and is encoded by a 1473 base transcript. The principal function of this protein appears to be as an autocrine regulator of p53. Induction of p53 induces transcription of the full length mdm-2 transcript, which is duly translated to the protein. The mdm-2 protein then complexes with p53, relieving the transient repression of cell replication imposed by p53 and preventing overaccumulation of wild-type p53 which might trigger apoptosis. Inactivation of p53 in turn effectively relieves the transactivation of the mdm-2 response element, restoring balance within the circuit. The fact that disturbance of this balance could dramatically effect the fate of a proliferating cell was rapidly recognised. Amplification and overexpression of the mdm-2 protein could override the halt normally imposed by the induction of p53 in response to genotoxic injury by blocking its transactivation domain, which effectively blocks induction of those products which are the effector arms of the p53 control circuit (Fig. 1). This includes those products which would lead to activation of apoptosis. Amplification of mdm-2 does not appear to be the sole means of evading the control which would be imposed by functional p53. However, amplification of the mdm-2 gene has been described in soft tissue sarcomas, malignant gliomas and anaplastic astrocytomas [45,46]. The role played by mdm-2 in other tumours has not yet been fully resolved. Amplification of the mdm-2 gene has proven to be uncommon in a variety of different tumours including Ewing's sarcomas, malignant melanomas, osteosarcomas, cervical and breast carcinomas. Overexpression of the mdm-2 protein has been found to arise as a result of gene amplification but may also be brought about by transcriptional and translational control mechanisms [47,48].

Although mdm-2 gene amplification in breast cancer has proven to be uncommon (5.4-15.4%), varied frequency of mdm-2 RNA and protein overexpression has been reported (13.8-38%) [49-52]. Using a commercially available antibody raised against an amino-terminal mdm-2 construct we examined mdm-2 expression in a series of 287 primary breast carcinomas in which nuclear IHC staining was evident in 20%. When comparing nuclear accumulation of mdm-2 with clinicopathological markers of prognosis in univariate analysis, positive correlations were observed with established indicators of better patient prognosis. A strong correlation was evident between nuclear mdm-2 immunostaining and low tumour grade (p=0.0181) (Fig. 4). In addition, correlations were observed between mdm-2 and steroid hormone receptor (ER and PgR) expression (p=0.073 and p=0.0125) (Fig. 5), reinforcing the suggestion that mdm-2 expression may also be regulated through these receptors [53,54]. No relation was observed between mdm-2 expression and c-erbB-2, Ki67 or nm23 expression, nor with incidence of axillary lymph node metastases. These observations contrast with other reports which have found associations between mdm-2 amplifica-

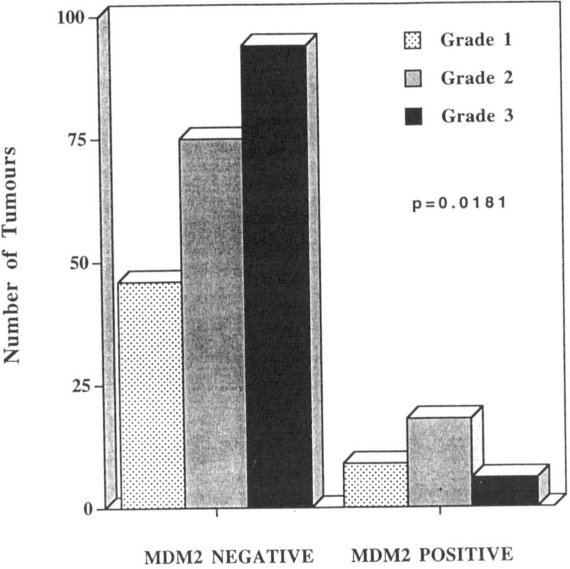

Fig. 4. Illustration of the statistically significant association observed between Bloom and Richardson high tumour grade and tumour mdm-2 IHC negativity.

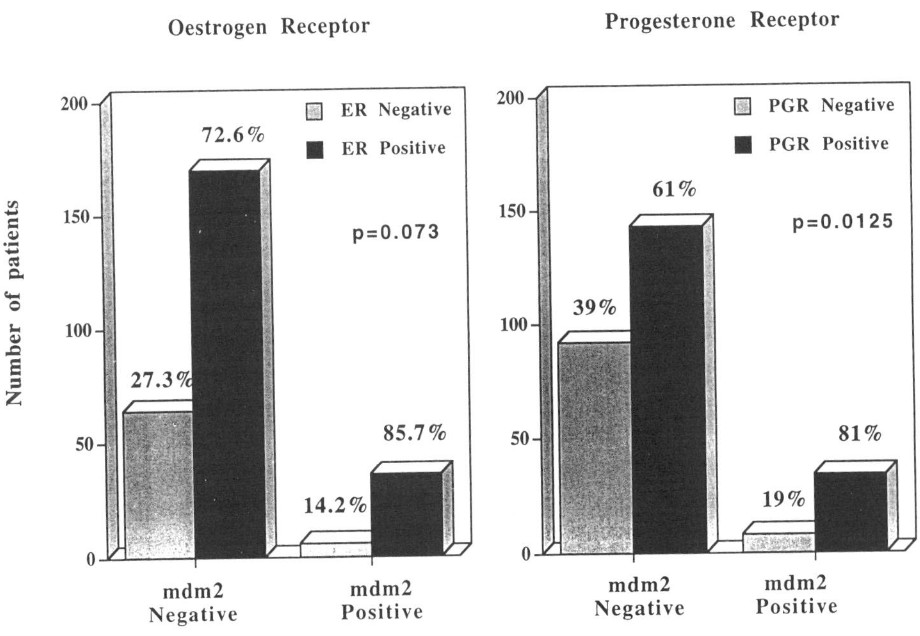

Fig. 5. Relationships observed between tumour hormone receptor expression and mdm-2.

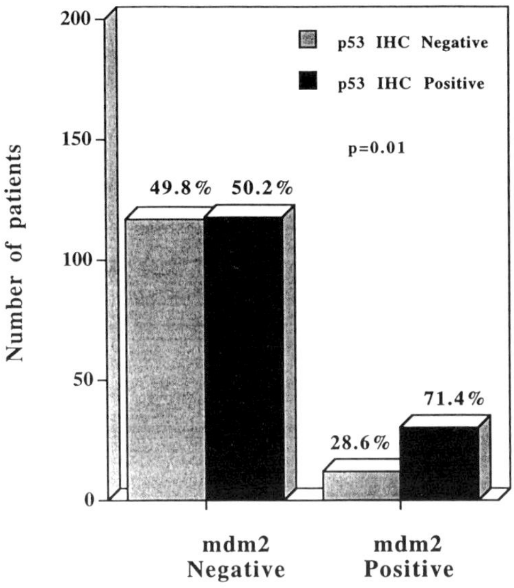

Fig. 6. Relationship observed between tumour nuclear p53 immunostaining and mdm-2 immunostaining.

tion, c-erbB-2 expression and late or aggressive cancers, as well as with angiogenesis [49,50,52]. Comparison of mdm-2 expression with nuclear p53 accumulation in our series of breast tumours, which comprises interval and screen-detected tumours, revealed a significant relationship (p=0.01). Of 148 tumours which were IHC positive for p53 immunostaining 30 proved also to be positive for mdm-2. This proportion of p53/mdm-2 dual positives represented over 70% of the mdm-2-positive group as a whole (Fig. 6). As IHC-detectable accumulation of p53 has been associated with mutation this observation is quite interesting since induction of mdm-2 is thought to be dependent upon transactivation by functional p53. Previous studies of mdm-2 protein expression in primary breast cancers which have used IHC to detect mdm-2 accumulation have reported marginally lower percentages of tumour expression but, in line with *in vitro* studies, have indicated that high mdm-2 expression correlates with presence of ER [51,53,54]. However, no other general positive correlation of p53 and mdm-2 expression in breast cancer has been described [55], with the exception of co-accumulation of wild-type p53 and mdm-2 in one sporadic tumour found to possess amplified copies of the mdm-2 gene and tumours from a cancer prone family [55,56]. In this latter instance overexpression of mdm-2 appeared to be independent of gene amplification and was not associated with induction of other p53-activated genes including p21. Thus it was proposed that the transactivational activity of p53 in this instance was at least in part inhibited by mdm-2, as would be the induction/repression of the genes involved in initiating apoptosis, thus accounting for the cellular tolerance of high levels of wild-type p53 and the increased susceptibility of this family to develop cancers. While this observation may describe the basis of a hereditary syndrome it does not account for the general observation made within our study population. However, the role, if any, played by mdm-2 in the genesis of breast cancer and other epithelial tumours may not be analogous to that assumed in soft tissue sarcomas.

The bulk of present research into the interactions of mdm-2 has concentrated upon defining the molecular basis of the binding between mdm-2 and p53, most recently with a view to designing appropriate strategies which could interfere with this process [44,57]. However, this work has been augmented by research which has begun to define the subtleties of the varied interactions of mdm-2 with proteins other than p53. Such reactions have recently been described between mdm-2 and the C-region of the retinoblastoma gene product (pRB), the activation domain of the transcription factor E2F-1, as well as the L5 ribosomal protein/5s RNA complex and specific RNA sequences, reinforcing the role of mdm-2 as a regulator of transcription [58-60]. The role played by mdm-2 in regulation of transcription and in the process of oncogenesis is further complicated by the recent observations that mdm-2 encodes not one but a family of a least six different transcripts (Fig. 7) [61]. Only two of these transcripts, the full length (1473 base) and the shortest mdm-2-e (249 base), retain enough of the NH_2-terminal p53 binding domain to complex with p53 when co-translated *in vitro*. All splice variants lack the primary nuclear localisation signal but a second such signal has been identified within the ring finger. Transcripts a & c retain the bulk of the acidic activation domain as well as ring-finger and zinc-finger putative DNA binding motifs, while others, namely b & d, retain the ring-finger and/or zinc-finger motifs. The biological significance of these different forms may well vary, as may their role in oncogenesis. The truncated forms lacking the p53 binding domain have been shown to induce increased transformation

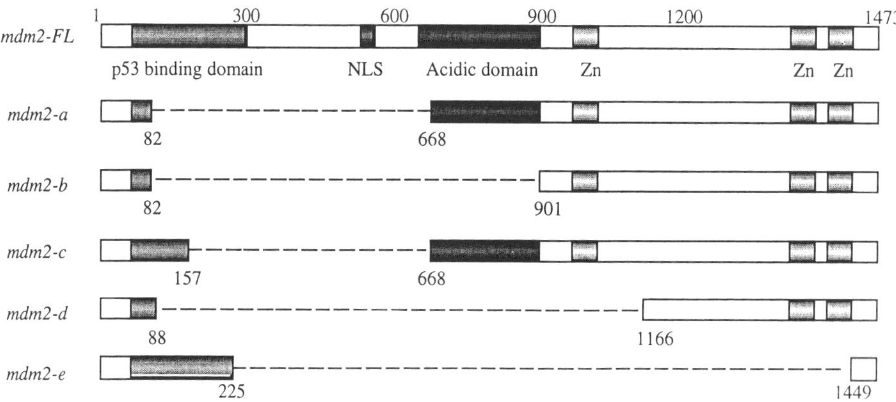

Fig. 7. Detailed maps of the multiple alternate spliced mdm-2 transcripts amplified from ovarian tumours. The illustration highlights the integrity of the principal functional domains of the variants in relation to the full length product. (Reproduced from [61])

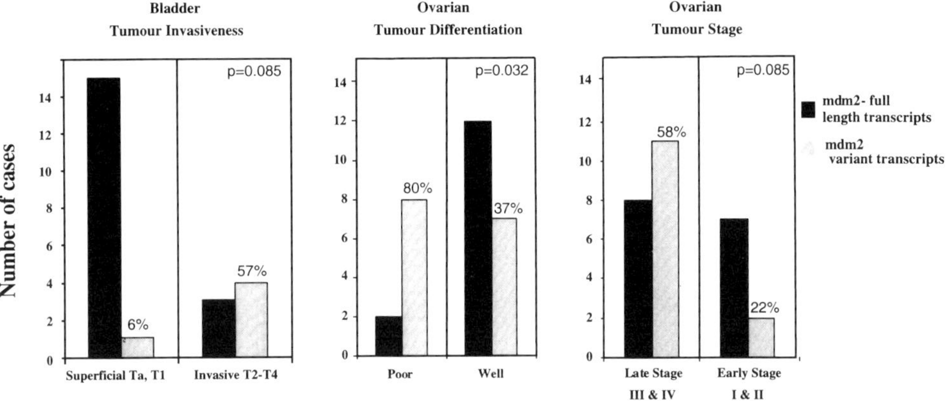

Fig. 8. Graphical representation of the association of the occurrence of multiple spliced variants of mdm-2 with tumour invasiveness, differentiation and stage. (Compiled from data originally presented in [61])

rates when transfected into NIH-3T3 Balb/c fibroblasts when compared with the full length product. In addition, occurrence of these multiple variants has been found to be significantly associated with invasiveness in bladder carcinomas as well as with late stage and poor tumour differentiation in primary ovarian tumours (Fig. 8). Multiple mdm-2 transcripts have now also been found in breast carcinoma cell lines, as well as in breast epithelium [54, and Lunec & Anderson, unpublished observations].

Conclusions

In general, it may be said that should estimation of p53 alterations be used to direct treatment upon the basis of likely tumour behaviour and outcome, the most reliable assessment could be made by combining molecular analysis of mutation throughout the entire coding region with IHC assessment of protein accumulation and localisation, which would be made with a number of antibodies. Such comprehensive assessment of alteration would prove expensive and depend upon adequately trained personnel and appropriate equipment. Unfortunately, for many smaller laboratories such an option may simply be non-viable, although together this combined estimation may further strengthen the value of p53 alterations as a marker of prognosis. However, if p53 alterations were to become more important as a directive factor that could predict responsiveness to cancer therapies, in particular those therapies which involve induction of the p53-dependent pathways of apoptosis, then the savings made by appropriately tailoring therapy may reduce waste, reduce unnecessary patient distress and help offset the costs of comprehensive laboratory assessment of tumour p53 status. In addition, research which has focused upon the interaction of p53 with mdm-2 has highlighted the importance of considering p53 as part of a dynamic integrated and multifaceted control network rather than in isolation. Greater understanding of the interplay within this system, the interactions of mdm-2 and the significance of the different variants of mdm-2 and their impact upon transcriptional regulation in relation to E2F, pRB, p53 and p53-dependent pathways, may offer further opportunities to predict tumour behaviour and identify new potential therapeutic targets. The study of p53 and mdm-2 and their interactions in the processes of regulating the transcriptional machinery of the cell as well as in the processes of apoptosis may yet be the source of further valuable discoveries in cancer research as we move to the new millennium.

Acknowledgements

Work presented as part of this report was supported by grants kindly provided by the North of England Cancer Research Campaign.

References

1   Lane DP. p53, guardian of the genome. Nature 1993; 358: 15-6
2   Soussi T, May P. Structural aspects of the p53 protein in relation to gene evolution: A second look. J Mol Biol 1996; 260: 623-37
3   El-Deiry WS, Kern SE, Pietenpol JA, et al. Definition of a consensus binding site for p53. Nature Genetics 1992; 1: 45-9
4   Thut CJ, Chen J-L, Klemm R, Tjian R. P53 transcriptional activation mediated by co-activators TAFII40 and TAFII60. Science 1995; 267: 100-5
5   El-Deiry WS, Tokino T, Velculescu VE et al. WAF1, a potential mediator of p53 tumor suppression. Cell 1993; 75: 817-25
6   Buckbinder L, Talbott R, VelascoMiguel S et al. Induction of the growth inhibitor IGF-binding protein 3 by p53. Nature 1995; 377: 646-9
7   Smith ML, Chen IT, Zhan Q et al. Interaction of the p53-regulated protein GADD45 with proliferating cell nuclear antigen. Science 1994; 266: 1376-80
8   Miyashita T, Reed JC. Tumor suppressor p53 is a direct transcriptional activator of the human bax gene. Cell 1995; 80: 293-9
9   Miyashita T, Krajewski S, Krajewska M et al. Tumor suppressor p53 is a regulator of bcl-2 and bax gene expression in vitro and in vivo. Oncogene 1994; 9: 1799-805
10   Miyashita T, Harigai M, Hanada M et al. Identification of a p53-dependent negative response element in the bcl-2 gene. Cancer Res 1994; 54: 3131-5
11   Wu X, Bayle JH, Olson D et al. The p53-mdm-2 autoregulatory feedback loop. Genes Dev 1993; 7: 1126-32
12   Picksley SM, Vojtesek B, Sparks A et al. Immunochemical analysis of the interaction of p53 with MDM2; Fine mapping of the MDM2 binding site on p53 using synthetic peptides. Oncogene 1994; 9: 2523-9
13   Bottger V, Bottger A, Howard SF et al. Identification of novel mdm2 binding peptides by phage display. Oncogene 1996; 13: 2141-7
14   El-Deiry WS, Harper JW, OConnor PM et al. WAF1/CIP1 is induced in p53-mediated G1 arrest and apoptosis. Cancer Res 1994; 54: 1169-74
15   Vogelstein B, Kinzler KW. p53 Function and dysfunction. Cell 1992; 70: 523-6

16 Elledge RM, LockLim S, Allred DC et al. p53 mutation and tamoxifen resistance in breast cancer. Clin Cancer Res 1995; 1: 1203-8

17 Horne GM, Anderson JJ, Tiniakos DG et al. p53 protein as a prognostic indicator in breast carcinoma: A comparison of four antibodies for immunohistochemistry. Br J Cancer 1996; 73: 29-35

18 Parkin DM, Pisani P, Ferley J. Estimates of the worldwide incidence of eighteen major cancers in 1985. Int J Cancer 1993; 54: 594-606.

19 Allred DC, Clark GM, Elledge R et al. Association of p53 protein expression with tumor cell proliferation rate and clinical outcome in node-negative breast cancer. J Natl Cancer Inst 1993; 85: 200-6

20 Cattoretti G, Rilke F, Andreola S, Damato L, Delia D. p53 expression in breast cancer. Int J Cancer 1988; 41: 178-183

21 Sawan A, Randall B, Angus B et al. Retinoblastoma and p53 gene expression related to relapse and survival in human breast cancer: An immunohistochemical study. J Pathol 1992; 168: 23-8

22 Martinazzi M, Crivelli F, Zampatti C et al. Relationship between p53 expression and other prognostic factors in human breast carcinoma: An immunohistochemical study. Am J Clin Pathol 1993; 100: 213-7

23 Yamashita H, Kobayashi S, Iwase E et al. Analysis of oncogenes and tumour suppressor genes in human breast cancer. Japn J Cancer Res 1993; 84: 871-8

24 Barbareschi M. Prognostic value of the immunohistochemical expression of p53 in breast carcinomas. A review of the literature involving over 9,000 patients. Applied Immunohistochemistry 1996; 4: 106-16

25 Elledge RM, Clark GM, Fuqua S et al. p53 protein accumulation detected by five different antibodies: Relationship to prognosis and heat shock protein 70 in breast cancer. Cancer Res 1994; 54: 3752-7

26 Jacquemier J, Moles JP, PenaultLlorca F et al. p53 immunohistochemical analysis in breast cancer with four monoclonal antibodies: Comparison of staining and PCR-SSCP results. Br J Cancer 1994; 69: 846-52

27 Bast RJ, Desch CE, Ravdin P et al. Clinical practice guidelines for the use of tumor markers in breast and colorectal cancer. J Clin Oncol 1996; 14: 2843-77

28 Visscher DW, Sarkar FH, Shimoyama RK et al. Correlation between p53 immuno-staining patterns and gene sequence mutations in breast carcinoma. Diag Mol Pathol 1996; 5: 187-93

29 Andersen TI, Børresen A-L. Alterations of the TP53 gene as apotential prognostic marker in breast carcinomas: Advantages of using constant denaturant gel electrophoresis in mutation detection. Diag Mol Pathol 1995; 4: 203-11

30 Deng G, Chen LC, Schott DR et al. Loss of heterozygosity and p53 gene mutations in breast cancer. Cancer Res 1994; 54: 499-505

31 Blaszyk H, Hartmann A, Tamura Y et al. Molecular epidemiology of breast cancers in northern and southern Japan: The frequency, clustering, and patterns of p53 gene mutations differ among these two low-risk populations. Oncogene 1996; 13: 2159-66

32 Hartmann A, Blaszyk H, McGovern RM et al. P53 gene mutations inside and outside of exons 5-8: The patterns differ in breast and other cancers. Oncogene 1995; 10: 681-8

33 Elledge RM, Fuqua S, Clark GM et al. Prognostic significance of p53 gene alterations in node-negative breast cancer. Breast Cancer Res Treat 1993; 26: 225-35

34 Kovach JS, Hartmann A, Blaszyk H et al. Mutation detection by highly sensitive methods indicates that p53 gene mutations in breast cancer can have important prognostic value. Proc Natl Acad Sci USA 1996; 93: 1093-6

35 Thorlacius S, Børresen AL, Eyfjord JE. Somatic p53 mutations in human breast carcinomas in an Icelandic population: A prognostic factor. Cancer Res 1993; 53: 1637-41

36 Sasa M, Kondo K, Komaki K et al. p53 alteration correlates with negative ER, negative PgR, and high histologic grade in breast cancer. J Surg Oncol 1994; 56: 46-50

37   Tsuda H, Iwaya K, Fukutomi T et al. P53 mutations and c-erbB-2 amplification in intraductal and invasive breast carcinomas of high histologic grade. Japn J Cancer Res 1993; 84: 394-401

38   Caleffi M, Teague MW, Jensen RA et al. P53 gene mutations and steroid receptor status in breast cancer: Clinicopathologic correlations and prognostic assessment. Cancer 1994; 73: 2147-56

39   Shiao YH, Chen VW, Wu XC et al. Racial disparity in the association of p53 gene alterations with breast cancer survival. Cancer Res 1995; 55: 1485-90

40   Saitoh S, Cunningham J, De VE et al. p53 gene mutations in breast cancers in mid-western US women: Null as well as missense-type mutations are associated with poor prognosis. Oncogene 1994; 9: 2869-75

41   Senmark-Askmalam M, Stal O, Sullivan S et al. Cellular accumulation of p53 protein: An independent prognostic factor in stage II breast cancer. Eur J Cancer 1994; 30A 175-180

42   Soong R, Robbins PD, Dix BR et al. Concordance between p53 protein overexpression and gene mutation in a large series of common human carcinomas. Hum Pathol 1996; 27: 1050-5

43   Oliner JD, Kinzler KW, Meltzer PS et al. Amplification of a gene encoding a p53-associated protein in human sarcomas. Nature 1992; 358: 80-3

44   Oliner JD, Pietenpol JA, Thiagalingam S et al. Oncoprotein MDM2 conceals the activation domain of tumour suppressor p53. Nature 1993; 362: 857-60

45   Ladanyi M, Cha C, Lewis R et al. MDM2 gene amplification in metastatic osteosarcoma. Cancer Res 1993; 53: 16-8

46   Reifenberger G, Liu L, Ichimura K et al. Amplification and overexpression of the MDM2 gene in a subset of human malignant gliomas without p53 mutations. Cancer Res 1993; 53: 2736-9

47   Otto A, Deppert W. Upregulation of mdm2 expression in Meth A tumour cells tolerating wild type p53. Oncogene 1993; 8: 2591-603

48   Landers JE, Haines DS, Strauss JI, George DL. Enhanced translation: a novel mechanism of mdm2 oncogene overexpression identified in human tumour cells. Oncogene 1994; 9: 2745-50

49   Courjal F, Cuny M, Rodriguez C et al. DNA amplifications at 20q13 and mdm2 define distinct subsets of evolved breast and ovarian tumours. Br J Cancer 1996; 74: 1984-9

50   Fontana X, Ferrari P, Abbes M et al. Etude de l'amplification du gene mdm2 dans les tumeurs primitives du cancer du sein. Bull Cancer (Paris) 1994; 81: 587-92

51   Marchetti A, Buttitta F, Girlando S et al. mdm2 gene alterations and mdm2 protein expression in breast carcinomas. J Pathol 1995; 175: 31-8

52   Inada K, Toi M, Yamamoto Y et al. Immunocytochemical analysis of mdm2 protein expression and its relevance to angiogenesis in primary breast cancer. Oncology Reports 1996; 3: 667-71

53   Baunoch DA, Watkins LF, Tewari A et al. Mdm2 overexpression in benign and malignant lesions of the human breast: Association with ER expression. Int J Oncology 1996; 8: 895-9

54   Guadas JM, Nguyen H, Li T et al. Drug resistant breast cancer cells frequently retain expression of a functional wild-type p53 protein. Carcinogenesis 1996; 17: 1417-27

55   McCann AH, Kirley A, Carney DN et al. Amplification of the MDM2 gene in human breast cancer and its association with MDM2 and p53 protein status. Br J Cancer 1995; 71: 981-5

56   Picksley SM, Spicer JF, Barnes DM et al. The p53-MDM2 interaction in a cancer-prone family, and the identification of a novel therapeutic target. Acta Oncol 1996; 35: 429-34

57   Chen J, Marechal V, Levine AJ. Mapping of the p53 and mdm-2 interaction domains. Mol Cell Biol 1993; 13: 4107-14

58 Xiao ZX, Chen J, Levine AJ et al. Interaction between the retinoblastoma protein and the oncoprotein MDM2. Nature 1995; 375: 694-8
59 Martin K, Trouche D, Hagemeier C et al. Stimulation of E2F1/DP1 transcriptional activity by MDM2 oncoprotein. Nature 1995; 375: 691-4
60 Elenbaas B, Dobbelstein M, Roth J et al. The mdm2 oncoprotein binds specifically to RNA through its ring finger domain. Molecular Medicine 1996; 2: 439-51
61 Sigalas I, Calvert AH, Anderson JJ et al. Multiple alternatively spliced mdm2 transcripts with loss of p53 binding domain sequences: transforming ability and frequent detection in human cancer. Nature Medicine 1996; 2: 912-7

ESO Scientific Updates, Vol. 1
Prognostic and Predictive Value of p53
J.G.M. Klijn, editor
© 1997 Elsevier Science B.V. All rights reserved

p53 Protein Expression in Human Breast Cancer: Relationship to Tumour Differentiation and Endocrine Response

R.I. Nicholson[1], J.M.W. Gee[1], L.T. Seery[1], R.A. McClelland[1], M.E. Harper[1], B. Holt[2], D. Barnes[3], J.F.R. Robertson[4], S. Pinder[5] and I. O. Ellis[5]

1   Tenovus Cancer Research Centre, University of Wales College of Medicine, Cardiff
2   Department of Urology, Royal Gwent Hospital, Newport
3   ICRF Clinical Oncology Unit, Guy's Hospital, London
4   Professorial Department of Surgery, and
5   Department of Histopathology, City Hospital, Nottingham, United Kingdom

Introduction

To date alterations in the human p53 tumour suppressor gene are the most frequent genetic change identified in breast cancer [1,2]. Mutations to the p53 gene occur in approximately 30% of invasive breast tumours and often result in the production of mutant proteins which have lost sequence-specific DNA binding [3-5]. Since wild-type p53 acts as a suppressor gene, maintaining the genetic integrity of the cell by preventing cells with DNA damage from further proliferation and promoting their removal by apoptosis, loss of p53 function is thought to play a central role in both cancer development and therapeutic response [3,6].

It is important to note that such mutated proteins often have much longer half-lives than wild-type p53 and accumulate in the nucleus of the cell [7,8], where as a consequence they may be readily detected by immunohistochemistry [1,9-11]. The sustained abnormal accumulation of the p53 protein has thus been used in many studies as an indirect indication of a mutational change in the p53 gene. Although in a number of tumour types there is generally an acceptable correlation between molecular (presence of a mutation) and immunohistochemical (presence of overexpressed mutated p53) analyses of p53 [9,10], mutations in the p53 gene have been identified which abolish p53 protein expression (splice site or nonsense mutations), therefore giving a negative immunohistochemical result. These types of mutations are found in 5-10% of cases. Con-

---

Address for correspondence: R. I. Nicholson, Tenovus Cancer Research Centre, University of Wales College of Medicine, Cardiff CF4 4XX, United Kingdom.
Tel.: +44-1222-747747, ext. 2485, Fax +44-1222-747618, e-mail: nicholsonri@cardiff.ac.uk

versely, it is also known that tumours can overexpress p53 in the absence of detected mutations in the coding region of the gene. This anomalous expression, however, is specific to tumour cells.

In the current study we review our published and unpublished data on p53 protein expression in a well documented series of primary invasive and locally advanced breast carcinomas in relation to a number of pathological, biological and clinical variables, including tumour differentiation status and response to endocrine measures [12-14]. Parallel studies have also been performed on a series of *in situ* ductal breast carcinomas [15] and primary invasive prostate carcinomas.

p53 in primary invasive breast cancer

Almost a decade has now elapsed since the first immunohistochemical report describing the presence of overexpressed p53 protein in some human breast tumours [16]. Of particular interest was the observation that prominence of the protein in tumour cell nuclei was associated with poor prognostic features.

A universal observation from studies employing immunohistochemistry is that the p53 protein is highly heterogeneous within the breast cancer population, ranging from essentially p53-negative cells through to those exhibiting high levels of positivity [12,17,18]. In a previous study using the mouse monoclonal anti-p53 antibody PAb1801, which recognises an epitope near the N-terminus of both wild-type and mutant forms of the human p53 protein, clear nuclear positivity was observed in 43% (62/146) of invasive mammary cancers [12]. No staining of normal breast ducts, acini or surrounding breast stroma was identified. The percentage of tumour cell nuclei staining in positive cases ranged from 5-100%.

Most studies to date have demonstrated an association between p53 protein expression and the histological grade of infiltrating ductal carcinomas [12,18, 19], the accumulation of p53 being associated with a loss of differentiated features of breast cancer. We have observed a highly significant trend for increasing p53 positivity and increasing histological grade of malignancy [12]. Thus while only 14% (3/21) of well differentiated grade 1 breast cancers were designated p53 positive in our own study, the figure rose to 55% (43/78) in poorly differentiated grade 3 tumours (Fig. 1a), with the high-grade cancers also containing the majority of tumours which expressed the highest levels of p53 immunoreactivity (>50% cell nuclei immunostaining; Fig. 1b).

Subsequent subdivision of the data by the individual components of tumour grade similarly revealed a statistically significant relationship between p53 overexpression and increasing grades of nuclear pleomorphism (Fig. 1c), loss of tubular differentiation (Fig. 1e) and increased mitotic activity (Fig. 1g), again with those tumours showing the worse prognostic features most frequently expressing the highest levels of p53 (Fig. 1d,f,h). The above relationships are, in part, reflective of the tumour type, with cancers displaying undifferentiated

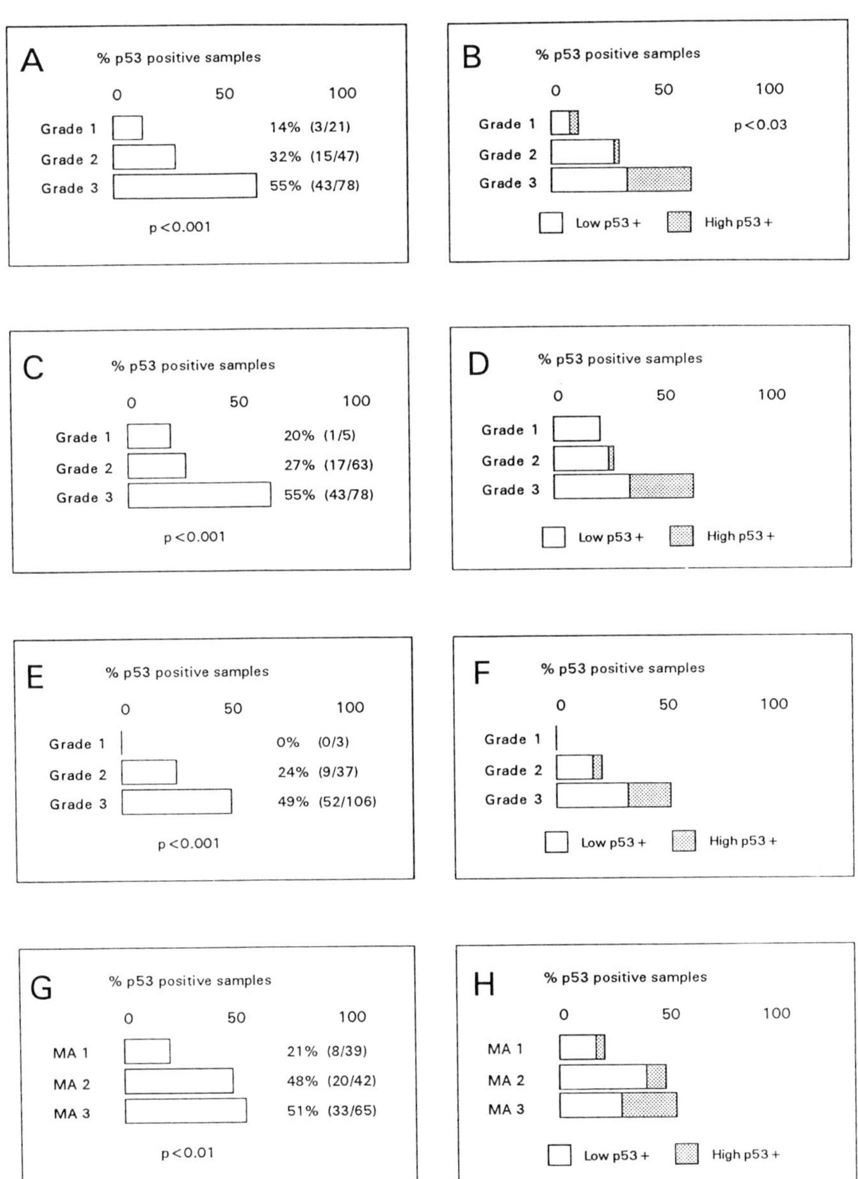

Fig. 1. Pathological associations of p53 in primary invasive breast cancer.
(a,b) Tumours were histologically graded 1 to 3 with increasing loss of differentiated features [12] and compared with p53 status and level as determined by immunohistochemistry. Data was further subdivided by the individual components of grade: - graded 1 to 3 with increasing (c,d) nuclear pleomorphism, (e,f) loss of tubular differentiation and (g,h) mitotic activity. p53 positivity was scored as high (>50% cell nuclei immunostaining) and low (5-50% cell nuclei immunostaining) in b, d, f and h. A chi-squared test was used to examine for trends.

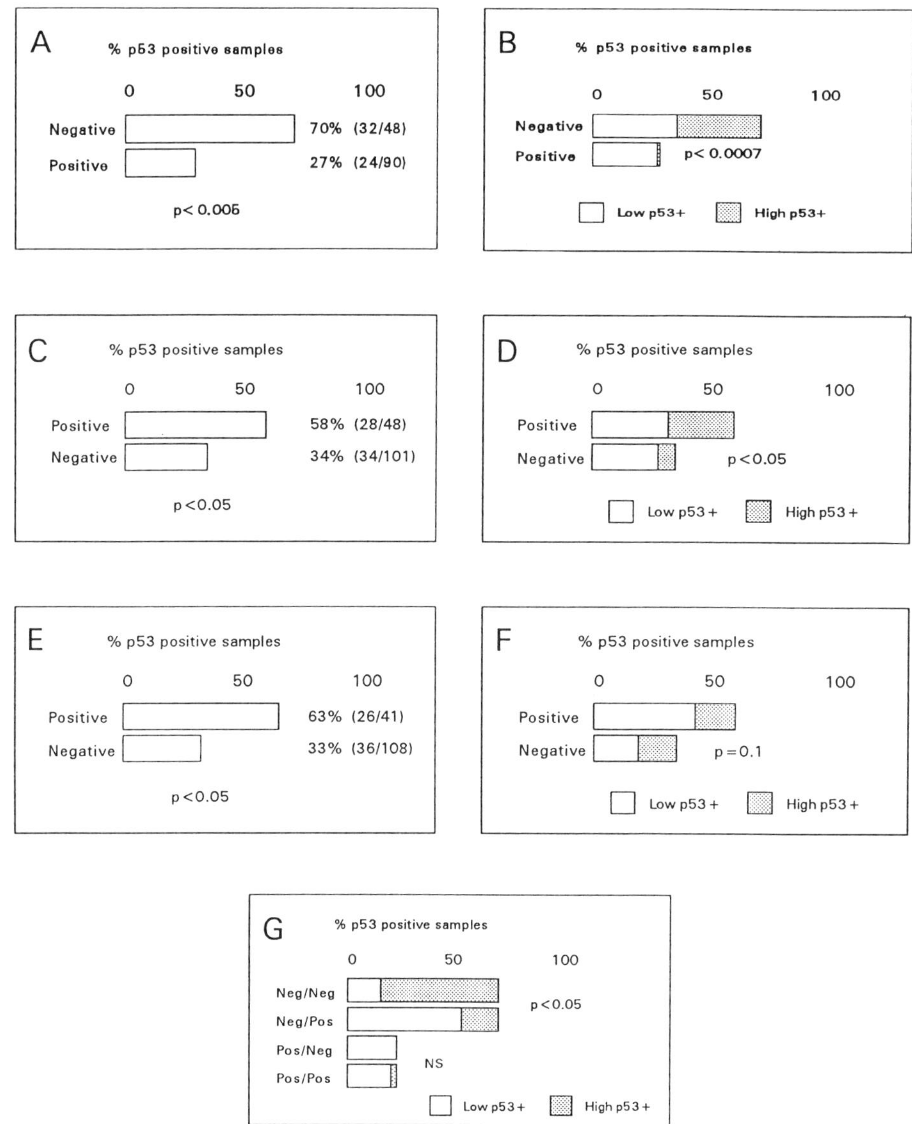

Fig. 2. Biological associations of p53 in primary invasive breast cancer. Tumours were assayed for (a,b) oestrogen receptors, (c,d) EGFR and (e,f) c-erbB-2 protein and compared with p53 status and level as determined by immunohistochemistry. In (g) ER and c-erbB-2 subgroups are shown. p53 positivity was scored as in Figure 1.

features frequently being classified as p53 positive. Thus while classic infiltrating lobular and tubular carcinomas are most often observed to be p53 negative, 60% of atypical medullary tumours were recorded as p53 positive [12].

In a number of studies accumulation of p53 has been shown to be associated with various other biological markers that indicate a poorer prognosis, including oestrogen receptor (ER) negativity and epidermal growth factor receptor (EGFR) and c-erbB-2 positivity [12,17,20-23]. Correlations between these parameters and p53 immunostaining status and level for our data on primary breast cancer are shown in Figure 2a-f and concur with the above studies. Of particular significance is the strong relationship between ER negativity and high p53 levels (Fig. 2b), with 16/32 ER-negative/p53-positive tumours showing the highest levels of p53 immunoreactivity, while only 1/24 ER-positive/p53-positive tumours fell into this category. Interestingly, in ER-negative disease, c-erbB-2 negativity also appears to be associated with higher p53 protein levels; 13/16 of such tumours showed the highest levels of p53 immunoreactivity (Fig. 2f) while the reverse was true for ER-negative, c-erbB-2-positive disease.

Although several other clinical features of breast cancer have been examined for their relationship with p53 immunoreactivity, including tumour size and lymph node involvement, no consensus exists in the literature. Previously, we have noted a non-significant trend for increasing tumour size and increasing p53 positivity [12]. In the current report this reaches significance if comparisons are made between tumours which are less than 2 cm in mean diameter (measured from the freshly resected pathological specimen) and those greater than 2 cm (Fig. 3a,b). In contrast, we have failed to observe any relationship between p53 status or level and lymph node involvement (Fig. 3c,d) or site of tumour spread (Fig. 3e), suggesting that the overexpression of p53 plays a limited, if any, role in directly determining the invasive capacity of breast cancer. This concept is reinforced by studies examining p53 expression in ductal carcinomas *in situ*, where an accumulation of the p53 protein has been observed in up to 25% of cases [15,24-26], that is, in tumour types which have not gained an invasive phenotype [15]. In our own study, positive p53 immunoreactivity (36/143 cases) was almost entirely restricted to large-cell, poorly differentiated tumours (Fig. 3f), a morphological subtype thought to be more inherently aggressive, and showed non-significant trends towards ER negativity and c-erbB-2 positivity [12].

p53 overexpression and prognosis

As stated earlier, immunohistochemical staining for p53 protein does not necessarily fully correlate with the presence of mutations in the p53 gene, nevertheless a large proportion of the studies examining its relationship with either disease-free survival or overall survival show a trend towards p53 positivity and worsened patient outlook [12,16-18,27-29]. Figure 4 illustrates this property, showing that the disease-free interval and survival characteristics of our patients with p53-positive tumours were significantly worse than those of the patients with p53-negative disease. Importantly, however, the prognostic effect of p53 is not large in comparison with other routinely assessed clinical and

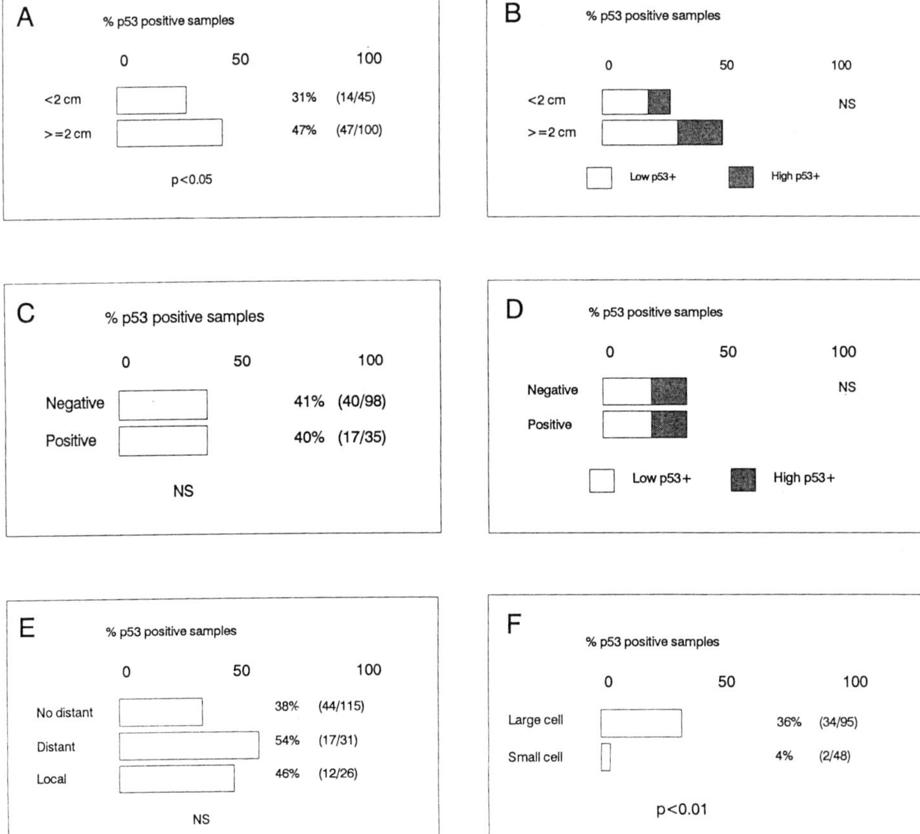

Fig. 3. Clinical associations of p53 in primary invasive breast cancer.
(a,b) Tumour size, (c,d) lymph-node involvement and (e) sites of tumour spread were recorded and compared with p53 status and level. p53 positivity was scored as in Figure 1. (f) Ductal *in situ* breast carcinomas were assessed for their predominant cell type [15]. p53 assays performed in the latter group were undertaken with the DO7 antibody [15].

pathological prognostic markers (i.e., tumour size, lymph node involvement and grade of malignancy [30]) and its significance may be lost in a multivariate analysis [1].

In the analysis of our own study group, p53 protein positivity was associated with a significant worsening of prognosis in lymph node-positive disease (Fig. 5b), while no effect was seen in lymph node-negative disease (Fig. 5a). This, however, is not a universal finding and the largest published study to date has reported a highly significant relationship between strong staining for p53 and poor prognosis in node-negative breast cancer patients [31]. Variation in the ob-

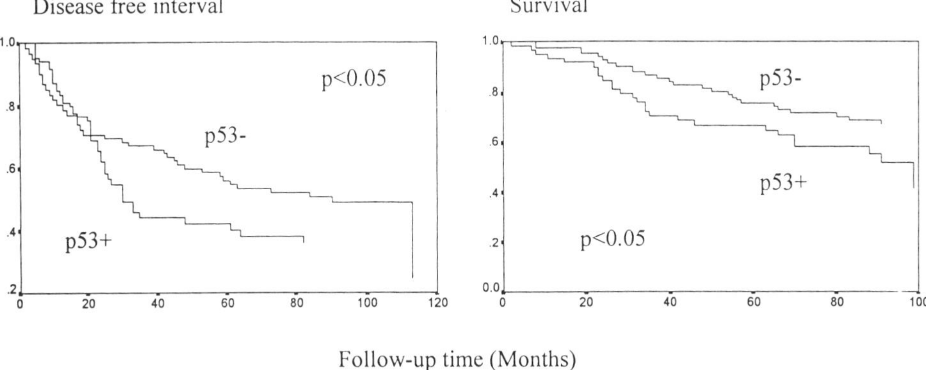

Fig. 4. Prognosis and p53 in primary invasive breast cancer. Probability of patients remaining (a) disease free and (b) surviving was calculated for patients in each p53 category using the life table method. Mantel's test was used to assess the difference between survival curves.

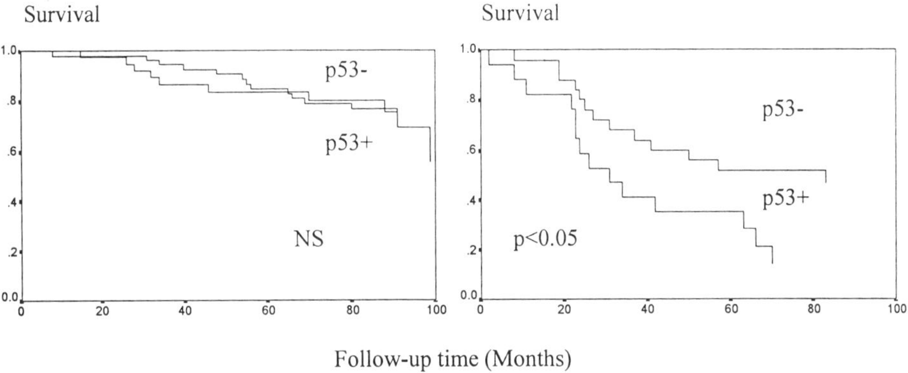

Fig. 5. Prognosis and p53 in primary invasive breast cancer. The results were derived as described in Figure 4 for patients with lymph node-negative (a) and positive (b) disease.

servations made above undoubtedly may reflect the relatively low numbers of patients involved in the majority of studies, differences in assay and staging/ grading procedures and variations in the distribution of mutated/wild-type overexpressed p53 protein levels [1].

p53 and endocrine response in advanced breast cancer

The pathways involved in determining the sensitivity of breast cancer to steroid hormones are complex and include ER interactions which induce cell proliferation and cell survival mechanisms [32]. Wild-type p53 is a known controlling factor for each of these processes [1,2] and when induced by antioestrogens it can directly activate pathways which inhibit cell growth and promote cell loss [33]. Blockage of the cell cycle by p53 takes place between the G1 and S-phase and involves the induction of p21 from the WAF1/CIP1 gene which in turn binds to cdk-cyclin complexes and inhibits the kinase activity needed for

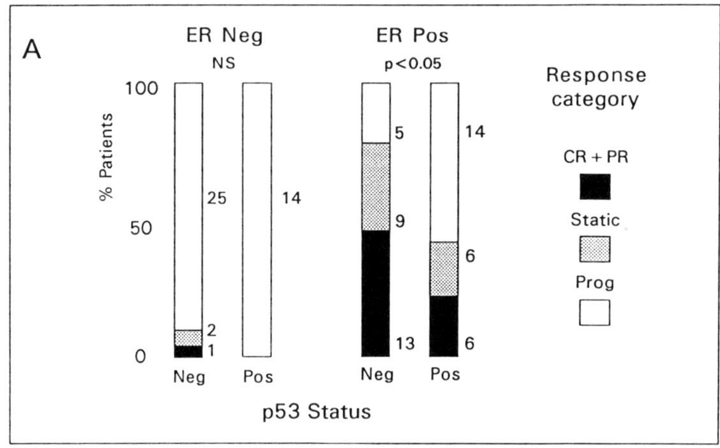

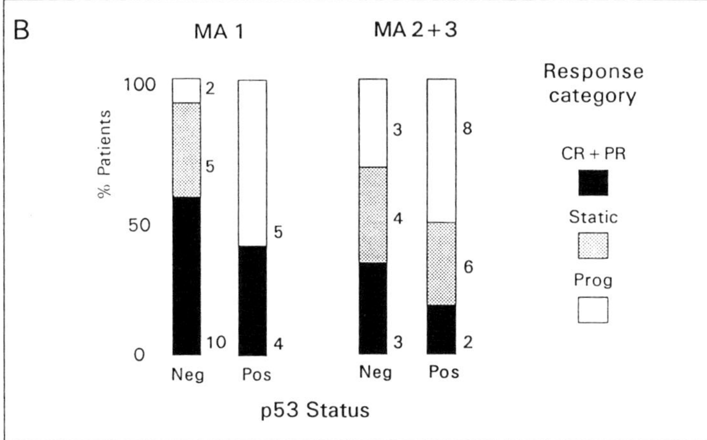

Fig. 6. p53 and endocrine response in breast cancer.
Patients treated primarily with tamoxifen were assessed for their response as previously described [42]. The results are expressed as the proportion of patients with p53-positive and negative tumours experiencing complete (CR), partial (PR), static (S) and progressive (P) responses. In (a) the data has been subdivided according to tumour ER status and in (b) by ER and a mitotic activity assessment (see Figure 1). p53 assays were performed using the CMI polyclonal antibody and only those tumours that showed positivity staining intensities ≥2 in over 25% of tumour cells were considered positive in the current analysis.

the G1/S transition [34-37]. Cells arrested in such a manner frequently undergo apoptosis, with the combination of cell cycle inhibition and induction of cell death instigating tumour remissions.

Loss of the above control mechanisms, through inactivating mutations in p53, may allow cells to proliferate unchecked in an increasingly efficient manner and to be more capable of surviving alterations in their growth regulatory milieu. In breast cancer cells it is envisaged that such changes may lead to hormone insensitivity or resistance to endocrine treatments. This hypothesis is consistent with clinical data relating overexpressed p53 protein levels with poor endocrine response.

Clinical responses to endocrine therapy for advanced breast cancer are observed most frequently (~60% response rate) in well differentiated, slow growing ER-positive tumours [38,39]. ER-negative disease is much more resistant to therapy and only 5-10% of patients show any clinical benefit. Figure 6a illustrates that in ER-positive disease the accumulation of the p53 protein is associated with a high failure rate to endocrine treatments (predominantly tamoxifen). Thus while only 5/27 (19%) ER-positive/p53-negative tumours failed to derive a degree of benefit from endocrine therapy, the corresponding value for ER-positive/p53-positive disease was 14/26 (54%). Such differences are reflected in the time to disease progression (Fig. 7a) and survival (Fig. 7b) curves for these groups of patients, with a significantly improved outlook for women with p53-negative tumours.

In parallel studies, the ER-positive tumours have been extensively examined for other biological endpoints, including EGFR [32,40,41], c-erbB-2 [40], TGF-alpha [42], c-fos [43] and bcl-2 [44]. Although in each instance the expression of these parameters has been linked to an aspect of endocrine response, their distribution generally did not differ significantly between p53-positive and negative disease. A significant difference was, however, noted between these tumour types with respect to the cell proliferation marker Ki67. ER-posi-

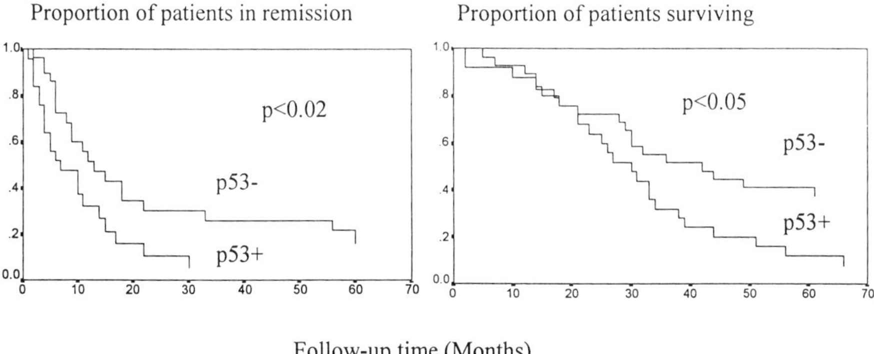

Fig. 7. Prognosis and p53 in endocrine treated breast cancer. Probability of patients with ER-positive tumours (a) remaining in remission and (b) surviving was derived as in Fig. 4.

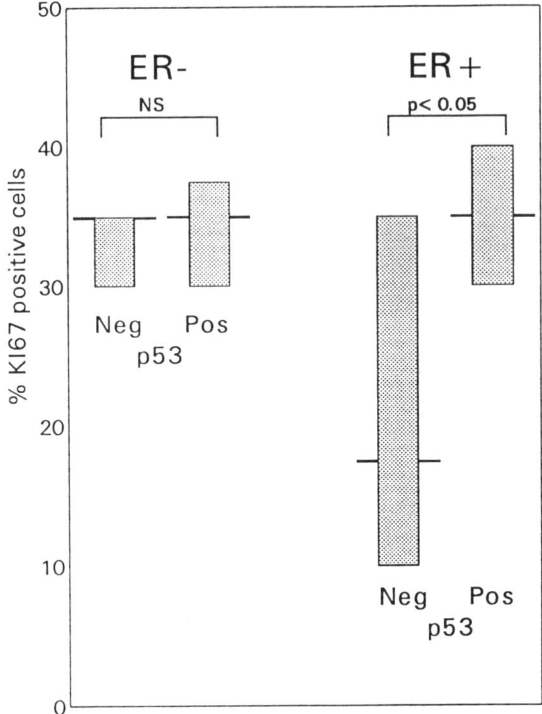

Fig. 8. Cell proliferation and p53. Tumours of known ER status were assessed for Ki67 immunostaining as previously described [45].

tive/p53-positive tumours show an increased proportion of Ki67-positive cells in comparison with ER-positive/p53-negative disease (Fig. 8), in good agreement with earlier reports where an elevated Ki67 score has previously been associated with an increased likelihood of failure to respond to endocrine therapy [40,45].

Interestingly, the presence of nuclear p53 immunostaining in ER-positive disease appears to be associated with an increased likelihood of endocrine failure, independently (to some degree) of the mitotic activity of the cancers (Fig. 6b). Thus, although indolent tumours show on average a higher response rate than those displaying more aggressive growth characteristics [40], p53 positivity is associated with a smaller proportion of endocrine responses in both proliferative and non-proliferative disease. Such data might infer that in tumours where p53 is overexpressed, the mechanisms which lead to endocrine failures contain an important component which is independent of the effect of p53 on cell proliferation; most likely the failure of mutant p53 to induce cell loss mechanisms. Further studies, however, are necessary to fully resolve this issue.

p53 in primary invasive prostate cancer

In a number of respects the growth and development of breast and prostate cancer are similar, both being reliant on steroid hormones, at least in their early developmental phases. Prostate cancer is, in most instances, slow-growing and most frequently presents in the older man. In common with breast cancer, it is treated by antihormonal measures, from which 70% of patients derive transient clinical benefit.

Surveys of p53 protein expression in primary invasive prostate cancer specimens removed by transurethral section have shown a relatively low positivity rate in comparison with breast cancer [47-50]; our own study unequivocally demonstrated positivity in only 19/90 (21%) specimens. Such tumours, like their breast cancer counterparts, are often drawn from poorly differentiated tumour types (Fig. 9a) which display increased levels of proliferation markers (Fig. 9b) and which are associated with a worsened outlook for the patient (Fig. 10).

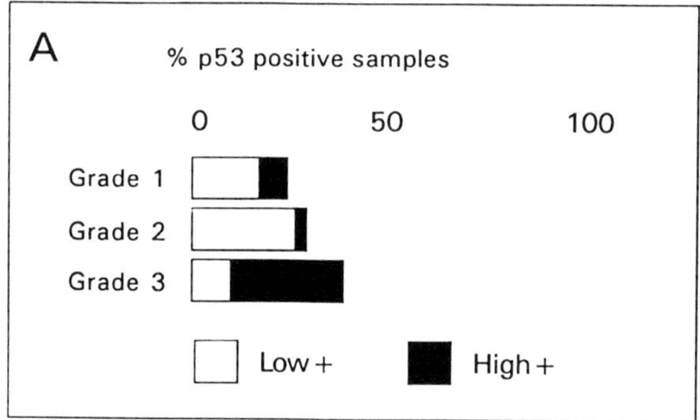

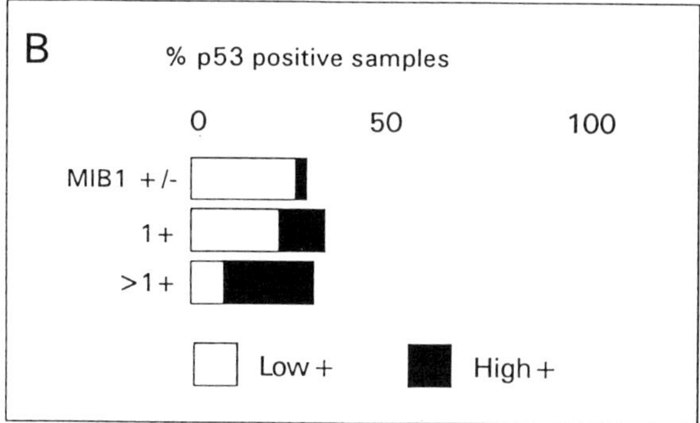

Fig. 9. Pathological and biological associations of p53 in prostate cancer.
(a) Tumours were histologically graded 1 to 3 with increasing loss of differentiation [51].
(b) Specimens were assessed for their proliferative index using the MIB-1 antibody [52].

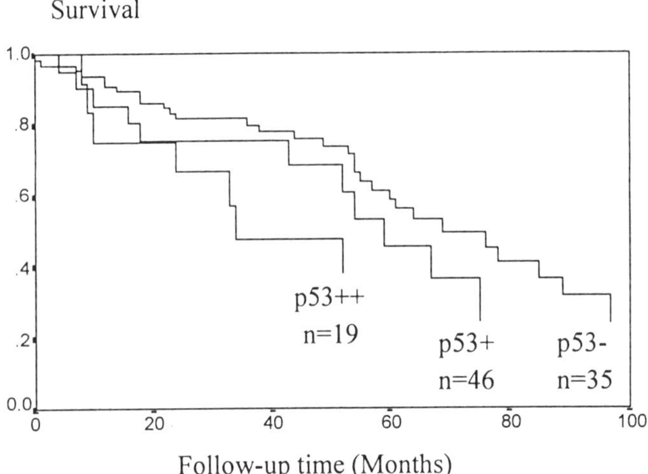

Fig. 10. Prognosis in endocrine treated prostate cancer patients. The results were derived as described in Figure 4.

Questions arising from immunohistochemical studies

The above data raise several important points worthy of further discussion regarding the role played by the p53 protein in the development of breast and prostate cancer and the consequences of its loss of function:

1. Is an accumulation of the p53 protein in breast cancer specimens directly responsible for the loss of differentiated features of the disease and its aggressive behaviour, or do p53 mutations merely occur more frequently in breast cancers which already possess a number of these features ?
2. Is it likely that alterations in p53 function are directly responsible for endocrine insensitivity and, if so, are these involved in the ensuing failure of endocrine measures to regulate cell proliferation and/or instigate cell loss mechanisms?
3. (a) Is an immunohistochemical approach in isolation worthwhile, can it ever fully define the spectrum of events arising from mutations in the p53 gene and (b) do aberrations in other elements of the p53 pathway contribute to the cancer phenotype?
4. Are similar questions also relevant to prostate cancer ?

1. Is an accumulation of the p53 protein in cancer specimens directly responsible for the poorly differentiated phenotype or merely a result of selection events occurring preferentially in undifferentiated cells?

Currently it is not possible to fully resolve these issues, indeed it is likely that they may not be mutually exclusive.

Normal p53 protein has been described as the "guardian of the genome" [53], a designation resulting from the central role that the protein plays in the cellular repair mechanisms involved in the recognition of, and response to, DNA damage. By blocking cell growth prior to DNA synthesis, and hence allowing for repair of DNA lesions, p53 helps to maintain the genetic integrity of the cell. In normal cells, if repair mechanisms prove insufficient, p53 also allows genetically impaired cells to be removed by apoptosis [54,55]. Normal p53, therefore, maintains the fidelity of the cellular phenotype by ensuring accurate replication of the genetic code. It follows from this that in cancers in which wild-type p53 is inactivated by allelic loss or by mutation, a cascade of genetic instability would be expected to ensue, readily facilitating gene amplification or deletion and changes in ploidy. Indeed, such changes would be further propagated since damaged DNA would not be efficiently removed from the gene pool by p53 -mediated apoptosis.

The net result of p53 mutations would therefore be to promote an increasing number of nuclear abnormalities and mitotic divisions, features which contribute to the definition of a poorly differentiated phenotype. In this manner, the inactivation of p53 would be expected to progressively generate more poorly differentiated features and an aggressive tumour phenotype. In addition to this, however, it is also likely that p53 mutations, in common with other genetic alterations, occur more readily in cell populations which already possess an inherently raised mitotic activity by virtue of an existing poorly differentiated phenotype. Such features are not only in place within the normal breast in undifferentiated basal cells, but are also present within the cancer cell population in the form of p53-negative yet poorly differentiated cells (Fig. 1a).

2. Is it likely that alterations in p53 function are directly responsible for endocrine insensitivity in breast cancer and are they involved in the ensuing failure of endocrine measures to regulate cell proliferation and/or instigate cell loss mechanisms?

To date, few clinical studies in breast cancer have directly addressed these issues and it is once again not easy to distinguish between p53 aberrations being causative of an effect or the result of it. Certainly, since p53 overexpressing tumours are often poorly differentiated and since poorly differentiated tumours are often endocrine insensitive due to an associated loss of oestrogen receptors [56,57], part of the relationship between p53 and endocrine response might be explained on this basis. Clearly, however, loss of oestrogen receptors is not the sole determinant of the relationship, since p53 overexpression also relates to endocrine insensitivity in ER-positive disease. It is interesting that these ER-positive tumours again tend to be poorly differentiated and what remains to be answered is what is the relationship between p53 and tumour differentiation/ endocrine response?

Possibly the most cogent reason for believing that alterations in p53 function play a role in determining endocrine response arises from its known cellular functions. Certainly it is well established that cytotoxic treatments, along with other forms of cellular injury, can sometimes result in apoptotic cell death in cells which have normal p53 function [58,59]. In contrast, p53-compromised cells treated in the same way frequently continue to grow and show little evidence of apoptosis. This has also been shown to be true for endocrine response in experimental models of ER-positive human breast cancer, where cells which are known to contain wild-type p53 not only show a lower rate of proliferation when deprived of steroid hormones, but also exhibit evidence of cell loss by apoptosis [33]. Aberrant p53 function is thought to compromise these events. Our clinical data in which p53 negativity correlates with i) low cell proliferation rates and ii) endocrine response, would also be consistent with a model where normal p53 function allows steroid hormone withdrawal to both inhibit the basal proliferation rate in receptor-positive cells and induce cell death mechanisms. Furthermore, aberrant p53 expression would lead to a less efficient inhibition of cell proliferation on hormone withdrawal, coupled with a failure to induce cell death. The net consequence of these events would be tumour progression, as observed in our study.

3 (a) Is an immunohistochemical analysis of p53 worthwhile, can it ever fully define p53 functions and (b) do other elements of the p53 pathway significantly contribute to the cancer phenotype?

(a) A consensus currently exists in the literature that the sole use of immunohistochemistry to detect aberrations in p53 functions is insufficient and that the technique should be combined with a molecular analysis of the gene to determine its mutational status. The combined use of these techniques could, therefore, generate information on situations where mutations/deletions have occurred in the p53 gene which fail to elicit overexpression of the protein and where wild-type protein is overexpressed in tumour cells in the apparent absence of mutations. Although insufficient data are currently available to fully address the biological implications of such changes, it is tantalising to speculate that some poorly differentiated grade 3 carcinomas which show no p53 overexpression may have, for example, lost both wild-type p53 alleles, while the small number of well differentiated tumours in which high levels of the protein are detected may overexpress wild-type p53. Certainly it has recently been suggested, albeit on the basis of very small patient numbers, that the overexpression of wild-type p53 may be associated with a good prognosis in women with breast cancer [60] and that certain mutations in the p53 gene may carry a worse patient outlook than others [61]. Such data, however, can only be confirmed or refuted through the use of a combined molecular/immunohistochemical approach directed at large cohorts of patients.

(b) In common with other important cellular control elements, the p53 protein acts to regulate complex downstream molecular pathways. It thus follows that changes in any component of these associated pathways may generate similar cellular consequences as loss of normal p53 function, or, alternatively, may provide an endogenous monitor of the occurrence of p53 genetic aberrations. Recently, an example of this has emerged from a clinical study of p21 (product of the CIP1/WAF1 gene), a critical downstream effector of p53 function which is inducible by the p53 protein and serves to block cell cycle progression by its inhibition of cyclin-dependent kinases. In this clinical study [62], patients whose cancers expressed both p53 and p21 (i.e. bearing either wild-type or a mutated p53 which is capable of inducing p21) had an improved survival in comparison with those whose tumours were p53 positive/p21 negative (i.e. bearing mutated p53 which fails to induce normal downstream effector events).

Of further interest is the murine double minute-2 (mdm-2) gene on chromosome 12q13:14, since its product is believed to be a transcription factor which binds to p53 and consequently abrogates its growth suppressing function. Overexpression of the mdm-2 protein leads to inactivation of the normal p53 protein [63], tumour progression and spread [64]. Amplification of mdm-2 is uncommon in breast cancer [63-66], while the protein is readily detected in the nuclei of a proportion of tumours [65,67], especially those which are ER positive [68] where it may even be under oestrogen regulation [68]. It is thus feasible that any significant increase in expression of mdm-2 in tumour cells may neutralise the actions of normal p53 and promote the same cascade of unfavourable genetic events as observed with direct mutations of the p53 gene [66].

4. Are similar questions also relevant to prostate cancer?

Nuclear p53 protein immunostaining in prostate cancer has been linked to increased tumour grade [69], tumour progression [70,71] and ploidy [69]. Unfortunately, however, no relationship has been conclusively demonstrated with survival or tumour stage [72]. Furthermore, the biological significance of p53 protein accumulation, notably its role (if any) in the control of proliferation and apoptosis in prostate cancer, remains largely unestablished. These latter factors have no doubt been influenced by the marked heterogeneous topographical distribution of anomalous p53 in the disease recently revealed by microdissection studies [73].

Importantly, however, careful analysis has revealed significantly more mutations in hormone-resistant prostate cancer than in its hormone-sensitive counterpart [47,74-76] and immunocytochemical analysis of prostate cancer specimens before and after hormone therapy has demonstrated a significant increase in the levels of p53 in post-treatment samples [76 and Harper, unpublished]. These data are compatible with the hypotheses that p53 mutations occur as relatively late events in the tumorigenesis of the prostate [47,50,75] and that their occurrence is associated with the eventual development of an endocrine-resistant phenotype [74-76].

Future prospects

Immunohistochemistry is an extremely useful technique which is capable of localising proteins to their precise cellular origin within complex tissues. The availability of a spectrum of antibodies recognising the stabilised overexpressed and/or mutated forms of the p53 protein has spawned a plethora of immunohistochemical studies examining a variety of tumour types *in vivo*. On careful review of the data, however, it is now evident that immunohistochemistry only represents the starting point for any assessment of the prognostic and therapeutic significance of p53. Although such studies invariably demonstrate a relationship between p53 overexpression and more aggressive features of cancer, too many anomalies exist between recorded protein levels and genetic changes to allow conclusive stratification of patients for treatment regimes. Therefore, while an immunohistochemical analysis of the p53 protein certainly gives us pointers to the role played by the p53 gene in determining growth responses within tumour cells (including the sensitivity of breast and prostate cancer to endocrine manipulation), future studies require a more thorough approach to p53 analysis, perhaps involving parallel genetic screening techniques.

References

1   Barnes DM, Camplejohn RS. P53, apoptosis, and breast cancer. J Mammary Gland Biology and Neoplasia 1996; 1: 163-75
2   Harris, AL. Mutant p53 - the most common genetic abnormality in human cancer? J Pathol 1990; 162: 5-6
3   Soussi T. The p53 tumour suppressor gene: from molecular biology to clinical investigation. In: Cowell JK, ed. Molecular genetics of cancer. Oxford, UK: BIOS Scientific Publishers Limited 1995; 135-78
4   Cho Y, Gorina S, Jeffrey PD, Pavletich NP. Crystal structure of a p53 tumor suppressor-DNA complex: understanding tumorigenic mutations. Science 1994; 265: 346-55
5   Hann BC, Lane DP. The dominating effect of mutant p53. Nature Genet 1995; 9: 221-2
6   Greenblatt MS, Bennett WP, Hollstein M, Harris CC. Mutations in the p53 tumor suppressor gene: clues to cancer etiology and molecular pathology. Cancer Res 1994; 54: 4855-78
7   Bartek J, Iggo R, Gannon J, Lane DP. Genetic and immunochemical analysis of mutant p53 in human breast cancer cell lines. Oncogene 1990; 5: 893-9
8   Varley JM, Brammer WJ, Lane DP, Swallow JA, Dolan C, Walker RA. Loss of chromosome 17p13 sequences and mutations of p53 in human breast carcinomas. Oncogene 1991; 6: 413-21
9   Dowell SP, Wilson POG, Derias NW, Lane DP, Hall PA. Clinical utility of the immunocytochemical detection of p53 protein in cytological specimens. Cancer Res; 54: 2914-8
10   Hall PA, Lane DP. p53 in tumour pathology - can we trust immunohistochemistry - revisited. J Pathol 1994; 172: 1-4
11   Wynford-Thomas D. p53 in tumour pathology - can we trust immunocytochemistry. J Pathol 1992; 166: 329-30
12   Poller DN, Hutchings CE, Galea M et al. p53 protein expression in human breast carcinoma: relationship to expression of EGFR, c-erbB-2 protein overexpression, and oestrogen receptor. Br J Cancer 1992; 66: 583-8

13 Willsher PC, Pinder SE, Robertson L et al. The significance of p53 autoantibodies in the serum of patients with breast cancer. Anticancer Res 1996; 16: 927-30

14 Archer SG, Eliopoulos A, Spandidos D et al. Expression of ras p21, p53 and c-erbB-2 in advanced breast cancer and response to first line hormonal therapy. Br J Cancer 1995; 72: 1259-66

15 Poller DN, Roberts EC, Bell JA, Elston CW, Blamey RW, Ellis IO. p53 protein expression in mammary ductal carcinoma *in situ*: relationship to immunohistochemical expression of estrogen receptor and c-erbB-2. Human Pathol 1993; 24: 463-8

16 Cattoretti G, Rilke F, Andreola S, D'Amato L, Delia D. p53 expression in breast cancer. Int J Cancer 1988; 41: 178-83

17 Horne GM, Anderson JJ, Tiniakos DG et al. p53 protein as a prognostic indicator in breast carcinoma: a comparison of four antibodies for immunohistochemistry. Br J Cancer 1996; 73: 29-35

18 Barnes DM, Dublin EA, Fisher CJ, Leviston DA, Millis RR. Immunohistochemical detection of p53 protein in mammary carcinoma: an important new independent indicator of prognosis? Human Pathol 1993; 5: 469-76

19 Pietilainen T, Lipponen P, Aaltomaa S, Eskelinen M, Kosma V, Syrjanen K. Expression of p53 protein has no independent prognostic value in breast cancer. J Pathol 1995; 177: 225-32

20 Dabbs DJ. Correlations of morphology, proliferation indices, and oncogene activation in ductal breast carcinoma: nuclear grade, S-phase, proliferating cell nuclear antigen, p53, EGFR and c-erbB-2. Modern Pathol 1995; 8: 637-42

21 Levesque MA, Clark GM, Yu H, Diamandis EP. Immunofluorometric analysis of p53 protein and prostate-specific antigen in breast tumours and their association with other prognostic markers. Br J Cancer 1995; 72: 720-7

22 Takahashi S, Narimatsu E, Asanuma H. et al. Immunohistochemical detection of estrogen receptor in invasive human breast cancer: correlation with heat shock proteins, pS2 and oncogene products. Oncology 1995; 52: 371-5

23 Visscher DW, Castellani R, Wykes SM, Sarkar FH, Hussain ME. Concurrent abnormal expression of erbB-2, EGFR, and p53 genes and clinical disease progression of breast carcinoma. Breast Cancer Res Treat 1993; 28: 261-6

24 O'Malley FP, Vnencak-Jones CL, Dupont WD, Parl F, Manning S, Page DL. p53 mutations are confined to the comedo type ductal carcinoma in situ of the breast. Immunohistochemical sequencing data. Lab Invest 1994; 71: 67-72

25 Leek RD, Kaklamanis L, Pezzella F, Gatter KC, Harris AL. bcl-2 in normal human breast and carcinoma, association with oestrogen receptor positive, epidermal growth factor receptor-negative tumours and in situ cancer. Br J Cancer 1994; 69: 135-9

26 Bobrow LG, Happerfield LC, Gregory WM, Millis RR. Ductal carcinoma in situ: assessment of necrosis and nuclear morphology and their association with biological markers. J Pathol 1995; 176: 333-42

27 Sawan A, Randall B, Angus B et al. Retinoblastoma and p53 gene expression related to relapse and survival in human breast cancer: an immunohistochemical study. J Pathol 1992; 168: 23-8

28 Isola J, Visakorpi Holli K, Kallioiemi O. Association of overexpression of tumour suppressor protein p53 with rapid cell proliferation and poor prognosis in node-negative breast cancer patients. J Natl Cancer Inst 1992; 84: 1109-14

29 Dowell SP, Hall PA. The p53 tumour suppressor gene and tumour prognosis: is there a relationship? J Pathol 1995; 177: 221-4

30 Haybittle JL, Blamey RW, Elston CW et al. A prognostic index in primary breast cancer. Br J Cancer 1982; 45: 381-66

31 Allred DC, Clark GM, Elledge RM, et al. Accumulation of mutant p53 is associated with increased proliferation and poor clinical outcome in node-negative breast cancer. J Natl Cancer Inst 1993; 85: 200-6

32   Nicholson RI, Gee JMW, Jones H, et al. erb Signalling and endocrine sensitivity of human breast cancer. In: Lichner RB, Harkin RN, eds. EGF receptor in tumor growth and progression. Berlin: Springer Verlag 1996; 105-28

33   Kyprianou N, English HF, Davidson NE, Issacs JT. Programmed cell death during regression of the MCF-7 human breast cancer following estrogen ablation. Cancer Res 1991; 51: 162-6

34   El-Deiry WS, Harper JW, O'Connor PM et al. Waf1/Cip1 is induced in p53-mediated G1 arrest and apoptosis. Cancer Res 1994; 54: 1169-74

35   Gu Y, Turck CW, Morgan DO. Inhibition of CDK2 activity in vivo by an associated 20K regulatory subunit. Nature 1993; 366: 707-10

36   Harper JW, Adami GR, Wei N, Keyomarsi K, Elledge SJ. The p21 CdK-interacting protein CiP1 is a potent inhibitor of G1 cyclin-dependent kinases. Cell 1993; 75: 805-16

37   Xiong Y, Hannon GJ, Zhang H, Casso D, Kobayashi R, Beach D. p21 is a universal inhibitor of cyclin kinases. Nature 1993; 366: 701-4

38   Nicholson RI, Gee JMW. Growth factors and modulation of endocrine response in breast cancer. In: Vedeckis WV, ed. Hormones and cancer. Boston: Birkhauser 1996; 227-61

39   Nicholson RI, Wilson DW, Richards G, Griffiths K, Williams M, Elston CW, Blamey RW. Biological and clinical aspects of oestrogen receptor measurements in rapidly progressing breast cancer. In: Paton W, Mitchell J, Turner P, eds. Proceedings IUPHAR 9th International Congress of Pharmacology, Vol 3. London: Macmillan Press Ltd 1984; 75-9

40   Nicholson RI, McClelland RA, Finlay P et al. Relationship between EGFR, c-erbB-2 protein expression and Ki67 immunostaining in breast cancer and hormone sensitivity. Eur J Cancer 1993; 29: 1018-23

41   Nicholson RI, McClelland RA, Gee JMW et al. Epidermal growth factor receptor expression in breast cancer: association with response to endocrine therapy. Breast Cancer Res Treat 1994; 29: 117-25

42   Nicholson RI, McClelland RA, Gee JMW et al. Transforming growth factor alpha and endocrine sensitivity in breast cancer. Cancer Res 1994; 54: 1684-9

43   Gee JMW, Ellis IO, Robertson JFR et al. Immunocytochemical localisation of FOS protein in human breast cancers and its relationship to a series of prognostic markers and response to endocrine therapy. Int J Cancer (Pred Oncol) 1995; 64: 269-73

44   Gee JMW, Robertson JFR, Hoyle HB et al. Immunocytochemical localisation of BCL-2 protein in human breast cancers and its relationship to a series of prognostic markers and response to endocrine therapy. Int J Cancer 1994; 59: 619-28

45   Bouzubar N, Walker KJ, Griffiths K et al. Ki67 immunostaining in primary breast cancer: pathological and clinical associations. Br J Cancer 1989; 59: 943-7

46   Nicholson RI, Walker KJ, Davies P. Hormone agonists and antagonists in the treatment of breast and prostate cancer. Cancer Surveys 1986; 5: 463-86

47   Aprikian AG, Sarkis AS, Fair WR et al. Immunohistochemical determination of p53 protein nuclear accumulation in prostatic adenocarcinoma. J Urol 1994; 151: 1276-80

48   Bookstein R. Tumor suppressor genes in prostatic oncogenesis. (Review) J Cell Biochem (Suppl) 1994; 19: 217-23

49   Dinjens WN, van der Weiden MM, Schroeder FH, et al. Frequency and characterization of p53 mutations in primary and metastatic human prostate cancer. Int J Cancer 1994; 56: 630-3

50   Grizzle WE, Myers RB, Arnold MM et al. Evaluation of biomarkers in breast and prostate cancer. (Review) J Cell Biochem (Suppl) 1994; 19: 259-66

51   Mostofi FK, Sesterholm I, Sobin LH. Histological typing of prostatic tumours. In: International histological classification of tumours, 1980, No 22. Geneva: World Health Organisation

52 Hepburn PJ, Glynne-Jones E, Goddard L, Gee JMW, Harper ME. Cell proliferation in prostatic carcinoma: comparative analysis of Ki67, MIB-1 and PCNA. Histochemical J 1995; 27: 196-203

53 Lane DP. p53, guardian of the genome. Nature 1992; 358: 15-6

54 Levine AJ, Perry ME, Chang A, et al. The 1993 Walter Hubert Lecture: the role of p53 tumour-suppressor gene in tumorigenesis. Br J Cancer 1994; 69: 409-16

55 Lane DP. p53 and human cancers. Br Med Bull 1994; 50: 582-9

56 Williams MR, Todd JH, Nicholson RI, Elston CW, Blamey RW, Griffiths K. Survival patterns in hormone treated advanced breast cancer. Br J Surg 1986; 73: 752-5

57 Robertson JFR, Dixon AR, Nicholson RI, Ellis IO, Blamey RW. Confirmation of a prognostic index for patients with metastatic breast cancer treated by endocrine therapy. Breast Cancer Res Treat 1992; 22: 221-7

58 Lowe SW, Bodis S, McClatchey A et al. p53 status and the efficacy of cancer therapy *in vivo*. Science 1994; 266: 807-10

59 Fujiwara T, Grimm EA, Mukhopadhyay T, Zhang W, Owen-Schaub B, Roth JA. Induction of chemosensitivity in human lung cancer cells in vivo by adenovirus-mediated transfer of the wild-type p53 gene. Cancer Res 1994; 54: 2287-91

60 Sjogren S, Inganas M, Norberg T et al. The p53 gene in breast cancer: prognostic value of complementary DNA sequencing versus immunohistochemistry. J Natl Cancer Inst 1996; 88: 173-82

61 Merlo GR, Bernard A, Diella F et al. In primary human breast carcinomas mutations in exon 5 and 6 of the p53 gene are associated with a high S-phase index. Int J Cancer 1993; 54: 531-5

62 Barbareschi M, Doglioni C, Veronese S, et al. p21/Waf1 and p53 immunohistochemical expression in breast carcinoma may predict therapeutic response to adjuvant treatment. Eur J Cancer 1996; 32A: 2182-3

63 McCann AH, Kirley A, Carney DN et al. Amplification of the mdm2 gene in human breast cancer and its association with mdm2 and p53 protein status. Br J Cancer 1995; 71: 981-5

64 Deng GR, He LW, Lu YY et al. Amplification of oncogenes HER2, mdm2 and myc in breast cancer determined by modified competitive PCR. Chinese Med J 1995; 75: 100-3, 127

65 Marchetti A, Buttitta F, Girlando S et al. mdm2 gene alterations and mdm2 protein expression in breast carcinomas. J Pathol 1995; 175: 31-8

66 Fontana X, Ferrari P, Abbes M et al. Study of mdm2 gene amplification in primary breast tumours. Bulletin du Cancer 1994; 81: 587-92

67 Bueso-Ramos CE, Manshouri T, Haidar MA et al. Abnormal expression of mdm2 in breast carcinomas. Breast Cancer Res Treat 1996; 37: 179-88

68 Sheik, MS, Shao ZM, Hussain A, et al. The p53-binding protein MDM2 gene is differentially expressed in human breast carcinoma. Cancer Res 1993; 53: 3226-8

69 Papadopoulos I, Rudolph P, Wirth B et al. p53 expression, proliferation marker Ki-S5, DNA content and serum PSA: possible biopotential markers in human prostatic cancer. Urology 1996; 48: 261-8

70 Stricker HJ, Jay JK, Linden MD et al. Determining prognosis of clinically localized prostate cancer by immunohistochemical detection of mutant p53. Urology 1996; 47: 366-9

71 Massenkeil G, Oberhuber H, Hailemeriam S et al. p53 mutations and loss of heterozygosity on chromosomes 8p, 16q, 17p, and 18q are confined to advanced prostate cancer. Anticancer Res 1994; 14: 2785-90

72 Brooks JD, Bova GS, Ewing CM et al. An uncertain role for p53 gene alterations in human prostate cancers. Cancer Res 1996; 56: 3814-22

73 Mirchandani D, Zheng J, Miller GJ et al. Heterogeneity in intratumor distribution of p53 mutations in human prostate cancer. Am J Pathol 1995; 147: 92-101

74 Navonne NM, Troncoso P, Pisters LL et al. p53 protein accumulation and gene mutation in the progression of human prostate carcinoma. J Natl Cancer Inst 1993; 85:
1657-69
75 Berner A, Geitvik G, Karlsen F et al. TP53 mutations in prostatic cancer. Analysis of
pre- and post-treatment archival formalin-fixed tumour tissue. J Pathol 1995; 176: 299-
308
76 Heidenberg HB, Sesterhenn IA, Gaddipati JP et al. Alteration of the tumor suppressor
gene p53 in a high fraction of hormone refractory prostate cancer. (Review) J Urol
1995; 154: 414-21

ESO Scientific Updates, Vol. 1
Prognostic and Predictive Value of p53
J.G.M. Klijn, editor

p53 and Angiogenesis in Neoplasia

Giampietro Gasparini[1] and Adrian L. Harris[2]

1   Department of Oncology, St. Bortolo Hospital, Vicenza, Italy
2   Medical Oncology and Laboratories, Imperial Cancer Research Fund, University of
     Oxford, United Kingdom

Introduction and biological background

p53 is the most widely investigated tumour suppressor gene and p53 inactivation/mutation has been documented with variable frequency in the most common types of invasive human cancers [1].

The wild-type p53 (wtp53) gene encodes a protein that inhibits tumour progression by complex molecular mechanisms leading to: i) maintenance of genetic stability; ii) stimulation of apoptosis; iii) cell growth arrest and differentiation and, ultimately; iv) suppression of tumorigenicity [2].

Recently, experimental studies have evidenced that wtp53 is also able to regulate angiogenesis. As normal cells progress toward the malignant phenotype, they must acquire angiogenic activity to attract and stimulate microvessel growth, and therefore p53 represents one of the first examples of genetic pathways regulating angiogenesis [3].

p53 stimulates the secretion of endogenous angiogenesis inhibitors

Our present knowledge on the molecular mechanisms by which wtp53 negatively regulates angiogenesis is mainly the result of a series of elegant studies performed by Bouck and collaborators at the Northwestern University of Chicago. Dameron et al. [4] demonstrated for the first time that in cultures of fibroblasts from patients with Li-Fraumeni syndrome (individuals who have inherited one wt and one mutant allele of the p53 gene and who have a high risk of developing malignancies when the wt allele is inactivated), the switch to the angiogenic phenotype is accompanied by loss of the wt allele of p53, resulting in reduced expression of thrombospondin-1 (TSP-1), a potent endogenous

---

Address for correspondence: G. Gasparini, Department of Oncology, St. Bortolo Hospital,
36100 Vicenza, Italy. Fax: +39-424-529880, e-mail: ggaspari@mbox.vol.it

inhibitor of angiogenesis. Furthermore, using transfection assays the authors found that p53 can stimulate endogenous TSP-1 gene, and that it positively regulates TSP-1 promoter sequences. These findings indicate that, in fibroblasts from patients with Li-Fraumeni syndrome, wtp53 inhibits angiogenesis by stimulating their production of TSP-1.

More recent studies by Stellmach et al. [5] indicate that wtp53 stimulates the secretion of levels of TSP-1 that are sufficient to maintain the anti-angiogenic phenotype also in normal mouse fibroblasts. The lack of wtp53 is capable, as a single genetic event, to induce an angiogenic phenotype in mouse fibroblasts.

The same group [6] found similar results in the BT549 human breast carcinoma cell line. The reintroduction of wtp53 inhibits tumour progression by mechanisms mediated, in part, through enhancement of TSP-1 synthesis and reduced angiogenesis. The transfected cells lost their angiogenic phenotype and became able to suppress neovascularisation induced by the parental tumour cell line.

p53 seems able to control the secretion of at least one other endogenous angiogenesis inhibitor. Van Meier et al. [7] have, in fact, demonstrated that wtp53 expression induces the release of an inhibitor of angiogenesis, called glioma-derived angiogenesis inhibitory factor (GD-AIF), in glioblastoma cells. This study shows that one result of p53 mutation during astrocytoma progression is the downregulation of GD-AIF and, consequently, the induction of the angiogenic phenotype.

p53 decreases the production of angiogenic peptides

wtp53 expression reduces by about 5-fold the production of endogenous vascular endothelial growth factor (VEGF) mRNA [8]. A study by Kieser et al. [9] on the other hand proved that mutant p53 enhances the production of VEGF in NIH 3T3 cells and promotes tumorigenesis, having a synergistic effect with protein kinase C in inducing VEGF-mediated neovascularisation.

A study by Dietrich et al. [10] shows that a protease inhibitor (N-acetyl-L-leucinyl-L-leucinyl-L-norleucinal) induces cell cycle arrest in platelet-derived growth factor (PDGF, a potent angiogenic factor)-stimulated human fibroblasts by inhibiting the proteasome. The authors found that the proteasome resulted in the accumulation of p53 which, coupled with an enhanced p21 activity, led to inhibition of activity of the cyclin-dependent kinase2/cyclin E complex.

p53 activity on vascular integrins and its effects on angiogenesis and apoptosis

Several adhesion molecules play a relevant role in angiogenesis and tumour cell invasiveness [11]. Among the adhesion molecules, integrins, immunoglobulin-like molecules and selectins are of primary importance in regulating angiogenesis [11]. The integrin $\alpha_v\beta_3$ helps endothelial cells to invade the extracellular matrix and enter the cell cycle, and in addition it is necessary for angiogenesis

[12]. Recent studies show that basic fibroblast growth factor (bFGF), but not VEGF, induces the expression of the integrin $\alpha_v\beta_3$ [13]. If ligation of this integrin to its extracellular ligand is blocked, vascular cells undergo apoptosis, which is accompanied by induced wtp53 activity, increased p21 expression and a decreased bcl-2:bax ratio [14,15]. These findings suggest a model in which the integrin $\alpha_v\beta_3$ plays a central role in regulating endothelial cell proliferation and survival in collaboration with p53 and other genes involved in apoptosis [11].

From the results of these experimental studies it emerges that wtp53 may influence angiogenesis in several ways, namely by: i) enhancing the secretion of endogenous inhibitors of angiogenesis; ii) suppressing the production of angiogenic peptides, and; iii) regulating endothelial cell proliferation, migration, differentiation and apoptosis with mechanisms mediated by specific integrins and regulated also by other genes.

Whether or not wtp53 regulates angiogenesis and which is the predominant molecular pathway involved, are cell type-specific phenomena [5]. In fact, there is evidence that, in general, the ability of wtp53 to regulate diverse genes and their associated functions may vary from one cell type to another [16].

Clinical significance of the codetermination of p53 and angiogenesis

Preliminary considerations on the clinical significance of the codetermination of p53 protein accumulation and angiogenesis as prognostic tools and as targets for novel therapeutic approaches in human solid tumours have been briefly summarised elsewhere [17]. Here we present an updated state of the knowledge in this field of translational research.

Breast cancer

At least six independent studies have analysed the prognostic value of p53 protein expression and angiogenesis assessed in the primary tumours of patients operated on for breast cancer [18-24]. In all studies p53 nuclear protein accumulation was assessed by immunocytochemical methods using specific antibodies (Ab240, anti-p53 protein MAb Novocastra and PAb1801). Similarly, angiogenesis has been assessed by means of specific antibodies recognising endothelial cells (anti-CD31 antibody, and antibodies to factor VIII-related antigen), by immunocytochemical methods, and by counting intratumoral microvessel density as suggested by Weidner et al. [25].

Horak et al. [18] studied p53 and angiogenesis in a series of 103 primary breast cancers (64 of which lymph node negative) followed up for 2.5 years, and analysed the reciprocal association and the prognostic value of the two variables for overall survival. Vascularisation was not significantly associated with p53 expression in either lymph node-positive or negative tumours. In univariate analysis for overall survival, when patients were stratified by the median vascular count of the series (100 vessels/mm^2), those with highly vascularised tumours (>100 vessels/mm^2) had a significantly poorer prognosis than those with poorly vascularised tumours (long-rank test, p=0.04). In this series p53 expression was not of prognostic value (p=0.80). Therefore, this pilot study, conducted in a heterogeneous series of cases regarding lymph node status, did not suggest any prognostic advantage for the codetermination of p53 and angiogenesis.

Toi et al. [19] determined both these biological markers in 125 breast cancer patients (57 of whom without axillary lymph node involvement) with a median follow-up of 5 years. The authors found that microvessel counts were not statistically associated with p53 expression. In univariate analysis for relapse-free survival, angiogenesis was significantly associated with the probability of relapse, using either the antibody to factor VIII-related antigen or the anti-CD31 antibody to stain vessels (p <0.01 for both). By contrast, p53 did not reach statistical significance for relapse-free survival.

A third study by Gasparini et al. [20] was similarly conducted in a series of both lymph node-positive and negative breast cancers (165 cases, 83 with lymph node-negative tumours, median follow-up 5 years). Using the PAb1801 monoclonal antibody to stain p53 protein, 28.5% of the analysed tumours were classified as p53-positive. No association was found between p53 expression and intratumoral microvessel density (highly angiogenic tumours: ≥80 microvessels/field). In univariate analysis both angiogenesis and p53 expression were associated with relapse-free survival and overall survival at a statistically significant level. However, in multivariate analysis for relapse-free survival, p53 expression did not retain independent prognostic value in a model including also cathepsin D, the joint variable epidermal growth factor receptor and S-phase fraction, tumour angiogenesis and nodal status. All these other variables significantly predicted the risk of recurrence in the multivariate log-logistic regression model.

The subsequent studies by the Vicenza group [21,22] and Costello et al. [23] were performed in more homogeneous series of patients because these studies analysed only patients with lymph node-negative tumours. Gasparini et al. [21] determined tumour microvessel density, p53 status and c-erbB-2 expression, hormone receptors and conventional clinicopathologic features in 254 consecutive patients with lymph node-negative tumours treated only with surgery and followed for a median time of 5 years. No significant association was found between angiogenesis (endothelium staining by means of the anti-CD31 antibody) and p53 expression (PAb1801 antibody used for staining).

In univariate analysis for both relapse-free survival and overall survival, angiogenesis and p53 expression were statistically significant prognostic indicators. In multivariate analysis angiogenesis retained significance for both relapse-free survival and overall survival, whilst p53 expression was statistically significant only for relapse-free survival. Furthermore, the patients with p53-positive tumours had a significantly higher likelihood to develop bone metastases than those with p53-negative tumours. The same group [22] confirmed these results in a subgroup of 211 patients of the same series by prolonging the period of observation. A novel finding of the re-analysis [22] was that p53 expression retained significance in multivariate analysis also for overall survival, which was related to the increased number of deaths among patients with p53-positive tumours compared to the initial period of observation [21].

Costello et al. [23] evaluated intratumoral microvessel density, c-erbB-2 and p53 status in a smaller series of 87 patients with lymph node-negative tumours, 37 of whom received heterogeneous forms of adjuvant therapy. No significant association was found between angiogenesis and p53 expression and none of the biological markers was significantly associated with prognosis.

More recently, Gasparini et al. [24] reported the results of the largest series published up to now of primary breast tumours in which codetermination of p53 status and microvessel density was performed. To validate the prognostic value of these two biological markers 531 patients were studied and followed for a median time exceeding 6 years. A subanalysis was separately performed in patients with lymph node-positive versus lymph node-negative tumours. In the final multivariate model, p53 status and angiogenesis were statistically significant prognostic indicators for both relapse-free and overall survival in the total series. In the subgroup of 260 node-negative patients, the final model of the multivariate analysis indicated that both p53 and angiogenesis retained prognostic significance.

As shown in Figure 1, p53 expression added significant prognostic information to the assessment of microvessel density. In fact, with an equal degree of

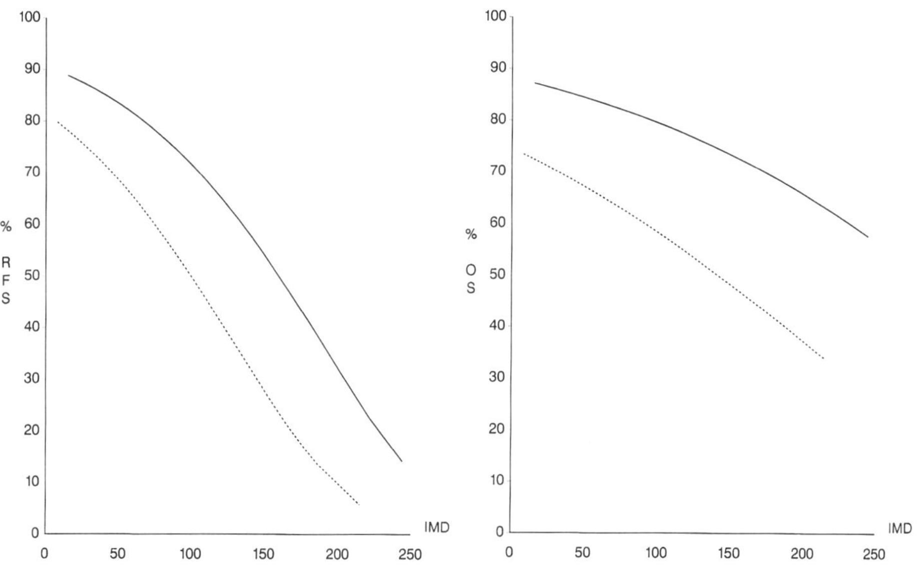

Fig. 1. Probability of relapse-free survival (a) and overall survival (b) of patients with No tumours. Intratumoral microvessel density (IMD) assessed as continuous variable and p53 expression assessed as dichotomous variable (- - - - = p53-positive; ——— = p53-negative).

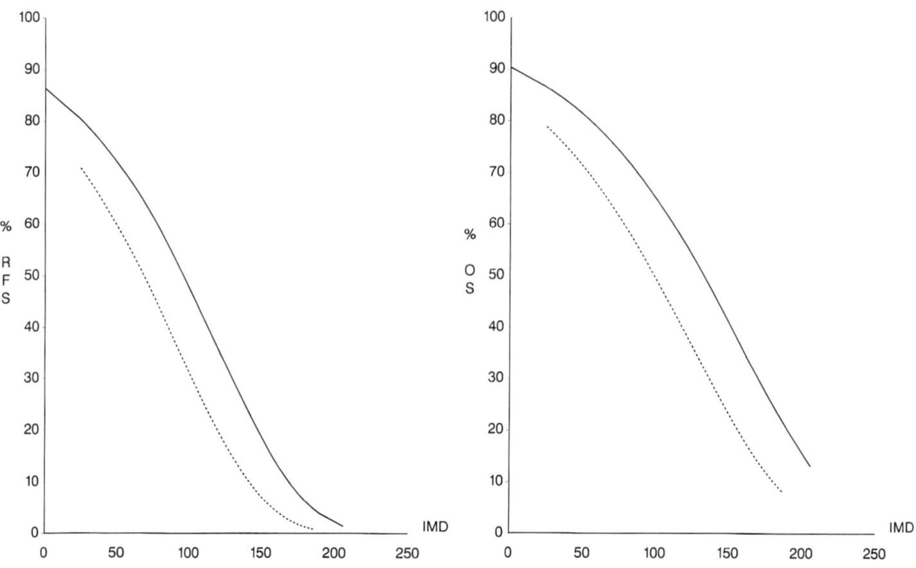

Fig. 2. Probability of relapse-free survival (a) and overall survival (b) of patients with lymph node-positive tumours. Patients stratified as p53-positive (- - - -) versus p53-negative (———).

vascularisation, patients with p53-positive tumours had a significantly higher risk compared to those with p53-negative cancers in this series. In the subgroup of 271 node-positive patients who received adjuvant treatments (chemotherapy: CMF schedule, or hormone therapy: tamoxifen), only angiogenesis and oestrogen receptor retained significant prognostic value in the multivariate analysis. The determination of p53 expression did not add relevant prognostic information in this latter subgroup of patients, as shown in Figure 2.

Overall, the findings of the studies reported here on breast cancer suggest that angiogenesis and p53 status are two independent biological variables, and that their codetermination seems to add useful prognostic information in the subgroup of patients with lymph node-negative tumours not treated with adjuvant therapy (Table 1). However, these results need to be considered with caution due to some methodological problems related to the assessment of angiogenesis and p53 using immunohistochemical techniques [26,27].

Other solid tumours

Two studies involving patients with locally advanced head and neck squamous-cell carcinoma have assessed the codetermination of p53 nuclear protein accumulation and microvessel density by immunohistochemical methods [28,29]. The first study [28] was designed to verify the association of p53 and angiogenesis with metastatic spread to locoregional lymph nodes or distant sites in a se-

Table 1. Codetermination of p53 expression and vascularity in breast cancer

Author [ref.]	No. pts.	Stage	p53 Marker	p53 Univariate Analysis RFS	p53 Univariate Analysis OS	p53 Multivariate Analysis RFS	p53 Multivariate Analysis OS	Vascularity Marker	Vascularity Univariate Analysis RFS	Vascularity Univariate Analysis OS	Vascularity Multivariate Analysis RFS	Vascularity Multivariate Analysis OS
Horak [18]	103	I-II	Ab240	ND	NS	ND	ND	anti-CD31	ND	0.04	ND	ND
Toi [19]	125	I-II	MAbNovocastra	NS	ND	NS	ND	anti-CD31	<0.01	ND	0.002	ND
								fVIII-RA	<0.01	ND	0.04	ND
Gasparini [20]	165	I-II	PAb1801	<0.01	<0.01	NS	ND	fVIII-RA	<0.0001	<0.0001	<0.0001	ND
Bevilacqua [22]	211	I	PAb1801	0.003	0.0009	0.025	0.036	anti-CD31	<0.0001	0.018	<0.001	0.044
Costello [23]	87	I	ND	NS	NS	ND	ND	fVIII-RA	NS	NS	ND	ND
Gasparini [24]	531	I-II	PAb1801	<0.001	<0.001	0.004	0.003	anti-CD31	<0.001	<0.001	<0.001	<0.001
	271	II	"	0.085	0.076	NS	NS	"	<0.001	<0.001	<0.001	<0.001
	260	I	"	0.003	0.003	0.008	0.016	"	<0.001	0.004	<0.001	0.03

NS = no statistically significant p value; ND = not done; RFS = relapse-free survival; OS = overall survival

ries of 70 patients treated with concurrent cisplatin and radiation therapy. Fifty-seven percent of these primary tumours were p53-positive, and in univariate analysis both p53 expression (p=0.04) and angiogenesis (p=0.004) were significantly associated with metastasis. However, in multivariate analysis only angiogenesis (p=0.01) and clinical stage (p=0.004) retained significance.

The second study [29] was conducted to assess the predictive and prognostic value of several markers in a series of 73 patients enrolled in a prospective randomised trial of concurrent chemoradiation therapy (cisplatin versus carboplatin and the same schedule of radiation therapy). Fifty-six percent of the tumours were p53-positive. p53 expression was significantly associated with high vascularisation (p=0.035), but not with bcl-2 expression. In this series p53 status did not predict the probability of response (i.e. clinical complete remission) to therapy. By contrast, in multivariate analysis both poor performance status and high microvessel density were significantly predictive of poor response (p=0.017 and p=0.045, respectively). As far as prognosis is concerned, p53 but not vascularisation was significantly associated with disease-free survival and overall survival (statistically significant level; α=10%). However, in multivariate analysis p53 retained significance only for disease-free survival, whilst vascularisation did not retain prognostic value for either disease-free or overall survival.

Recently, Gasparini et al. [30] assessed the prognostic and predictive value of vascularisation in a series of 60 cases with FIGO stage III-IV ovarian cancer. The authors found that in multivariate analysis, angiogenesis and performance status (p=0.01 for both) were significantly associated with pathological complete response to first-line cisplatin-based combined chemotherapy. However, vascularisation was not associated with overall survival. In a subgroup of 44 cases of the above series, also p53 protein accumulation was assessed (PAb1801 antibody). Sixty-six percent of the ovarian cancers were classified as p53-positive and a significant association was found between p53 expression and angiogenesis (p=0.025). In this series p53 protein was also significantly associated with histological grade (p=0.001) and cell proliferative activity (MIB-1 antibody, p=0.015). Angiogenesis, but not p53 status, was significantly associated with pathological complete response to chemotherapy. By contrast, p53 protein but not angiogenesis was significantly associated with overall survival in both univariate and multivariate analysis (p=0.03 and p=0.01, respectively) [Gasparini et al., unpublished results].

Bochner et al. [31] analysed the prognostic value of the codetermination of p53 nuclear protein accumulation and angiogenesis in a series of 126 patients with invasive transitional-cell carcinoma of the bladder. p53 was assessed by immunohistochemistry and it was significantly associated with high vascularisation (p=0.05). Both p53 status and microvessel density were significantly associated with disease recurrence and overall survival in univariate and multivariate analysis. In a larger series the same authors confirmed that angiogenesis is an independent prognostic factor in invasive bladder cancer [32]. However, in their final report [32] they did not report data on p53 status.

The results of another elegant study on translational research have recently been reported [33]; this study included a series of 163 patients with invasive carcinoma of the bladder. The authors determined microvessel density, p53 protein alterations and the expression of TSP-1 (monoclonal antibody MA-II), and documented that low TSP-1 expression in tumours is associated with p53 expression and high vascularisation. These results are in accordance with experimental studies showing that p53 regulates angiogenesis by modulating the levels of TSP-1 [4-6]. Furthermore, patients with low TSP-1 expression had a significantly higher probability of recurrence and death than those with tumours characterised by high TSP-1 expression. TSP-1 retained significance in multivariate analysis for disease-free survival and overall survival in a model including also tumour stage, node status and histological grade. However, TSP-1 was not independent of p53 expression.

O'Brien et al. [34] studied the expression of the angiogenic factor thymidine phosphorylase (TP), tumour vascularity, ploidy, p53 protein expression and conventional clinicopathological parameters in 105 bladder cancers. TP expression of tumour cells was significantly correlated with malignancy, invasive tumour stages, histological type and tumour grade. No association of TP expression with the other biological variables was observed. Regarding the prognosis of this series of patients, neither TP nor vascularity were of prognostic value, but patients with p53-positive tumours had a higher probability of death than those with p53-negative tumours, although the difference was not statistically significant (p=0.06). The authors concluded that TP determination is not a promising prognostic tool, but it may be a target of efficacy of therapy with 5-fluorouracil and methotrexate because TP catalyzes the reversible breakdown of thymidine to thymine, a biochemical step involved in activation of these cytotoxic drugs.

Two independent groups analysed the codetermination of p53 status and angiogenesis in non-small cell lung cancer patients [35,36]. Giatromanolaki et al. [35] studied 107 cases with operable ($T_{1,2}$-$N_{0,1}M_0$) non-small cell lung carcinomas using the antibody anti-CD31 to stain microvessels and assessing vascular grade with the Chalkley score. p53 was assessed by the polyclonal antibody CM-1 and immunohistochemistry. Fifty-five percent of the tumours were p53 positive and p53 status was not significantly associated with the degree of vascularisation in this series (p=0.30). Furthermore, vascular grade (p=0.0001), but not p53 (p=0.30) was significantly associated with lymph node metastasis. In univariate and multivariate analysis (in the model without N-stage) angiogenesis, but not p53, was of prognostic value (median follow-up 45 months).

Fontanini et al. [36] studied p53 status (PAb1801 antibody), microvessel density (CD34 antibody) and expression of VEGF (Santa Cruz Biochem. polyclonal antibody) in 73 patients with stage I-II non-small cell cancers, median follow-up of 47 months. The authors found a highly statistical association of p53 nuclear accumulation (p53 positivity in 68% of the tumours) with microvessel counts (p=0.0003) and VEGF expression (p=0.02). In univariate analysis p53 status and microvessel counts were significantly associated with lymph node

Table 2. Codetermination of p53 expression and vascularity in solid tumours other than breast cancer

Author [ref.]	Tumour type	No. pts	Stage	Marker	p53 Univariate Analysis RFS	p53 Univariate Analysis OS	p53 Multivariate Analysis RFS	p53 Multivariate Analysis OS	Marker	Vascularity Univariate Analysis RFS	Vascularity Univariate Analysis OS	Vascularity Multivariate Analysis RFS	Vascularity Multivariate Analysis OS
Gasparini [28]	H&N	70	II-III-IV	PAb1801	0.04**	ND	NS**	ND	anti-CD31	0.0046**	ND	0.01	ND
Gasparini [29]	H&N	73	II-III-IV	PAb1801	0.09	0.08	0.04	NS	anti-CD31	NS	NS	NS	NS
Gasparini*	Ovarian	44	III-IV	PAb1801	NS	NS	ND	ND	anti-CD31	NS	NS	ND	ND
Bochner [30]	Bladder	126	Invasive	ND	0.0001	0.0001	<0.05	<0.05	CD34	0.004	0.0001	<0.05	<0.05
Grossfeld [33]	Bladder	163	Invasive	PAb1801	<0.05	<0.05	<0.05	<0.05	CD34	<0.05	<0.05	NS	NS
O'Brien [34]	Bladder	105	Superficial and invasive	PAb1801	0.06	NS	ND	ND	anti-CD31	NS	NS	ND	ND
Giatromano-laki [35]	Non-small cell lung	107	I-II	CM-1	ND	NS	ND	NS	anti-CD31	ND	0.0004	ND	0.007
Fontanini [36]	Non-small cell lung	73	I-II	PAb1801	<0.05	<0.05	NS	NS	CD34	<0.05	<0.05	0.0009	0.0001
Vermeulen [37]	Colorectal	42	Dukes' B-C-D	D07	ND	ND	ND	ND	anti-CD31	ND	ND	ND	ND

*= unpublished results; ** = association with metastasis; NS = no statistically significant p value; ND = not done; RFS = relapse-free survival; OS = overall survival.

metastases, disease-free survival and overall survival. However, in multivariate analysis only angiogenesis and node status retained significance for disease-free survival (p=0.0001 and p=0.03, respectively) and overall survival (p=0.0009 and p=0.01, respectively).

Vermeulen et al. [37] studied p53 expression and microvessel density in a series of 42 cases with colorectal adenocarcinoma. Sixty-five percent of the cancers were classified as p53-positive. p53-positivity was associated with a significantly higher microvessel density (p=0.04). Table 2 summarizes the results of these studies.

Finally, Pezzella et al. [38] evaluated the expression of several markers including bcl-2, Ki67 and hormone receptors as well as vascularisation (anti-CD31 antibody, Chalkley score counting the three "hottest" spots/each tumour) and p53 protein (PAb1801 antibody) in a series of 36 solitary lung metastases from different primary tumour types (breast, 15; colorectal, 13; kidney, 3; melanoma, 3; other, 2). Overall, 10 metastases were classified as p53 positive. The median value of vascularisation was similar in p53-positive metastases (n=23; range 12-32) and p53-negative metastases (n=23; range 12-45).

Conclusions

Association between p53 protein nuclear accumulation and microvessel counts

The association between these two variables seems to be related to the tumour type in which codetermination is performed.

In invasive early-stage breast carcinoma, the range of p53 positivity was quite high among the studies analysed (from 22% [21] to 55% [18]), largely dependent on the heterogeneity of the series, the different antibodies used and the diverse criteria adopted to classify a tumour as p53-positive. In any case, in all studies reported here no association was observed between microvessel density and p53 protein expression when assessed by immunohistochemical methods.

In head and neck locally advanced squamous-cell carcinoma the frequency of p53 positivity (56% and 57%) [28,29] was considerably higher than that found in breast cancer and it was significantly associated with highly angiogenic tumours [28,29]. Similarly, the reports by Bochner et al. [31] and Grossfeld et al. [33] but not the one by O'Brien et al. [34] show a significant association of p53 status with microvessel density in invasive bladder cancer.

More limited and controversial are the results in non-small cell lung cancer. In one study [35] no association was found between the two biological markers, while in another study by Fontanini et al. [36] a significant association was reported. An interesting finding is that Fontanini et al. found a higher frequency of p53 positivity than the other study. Finally, Vermeulen et al. [37] found a significant association between p53 and angiogenesis in the first published study reporting the codetermination of these two variables in colorectal cancer.

Does codetermination of p53 and angiogenesis add useful clinical information to the assessment of each variable individually?

As far as breast cancer is concerned, the studies by Gasparini et al. [21,22,24] suggest that in the subgroup of node-negative patients not treated with adjuvant therapy, microvessel density and p53 are independent prognostic indicators. Therefore, the combined assessment of the two variables seems to be useful to increase the probability of identifying subgroups of patients at different risk of recurrence and death. Conversely, the findings of the majority of studies conducted in node-positive or mixed (node-positive and node-negative) series indicate that p53, in general, does not retain a significant prognostic value when angiogenesis is also assessed and included in multivariate analysis.

In head and neck cancer, the determination of p53 is of prognostic value but it is not predictive of response to treatment with combined chemo-radiotherapy. Angiogenesis, on the other hand, is predictive of response but does not have prognostic value [29]. Similar findings have been observed in FIGO stage III-IV ovarian cancer regarding the prediction of response to first-line chemotherapy and prognosis [Gasparini et al., unpublished results].

Also in bladder cancer one preliminary study [31] suggests that, like in node-negative breast cancer, p53 and microvessel density are independent prognostic indicators. However, another study performed by Grossfeld et al. [33] determining TSP-1, p53 expression and vascularisation showed that TSP-1 and microvessel density do not retain significance when p53 is considered in the multivariate analysis.

Finally, two studies reporting data on the codetermination of p53 and microvessel counts in non-small cell lung cancer showed that angiogenesis, but not p53, retained prognostic significance in multivariate analysis [35,36].

Based on these preliminary results, further studies on the codetermination of these two biological variables should be conducted in larger series of node-negative breast cancer, bladder cancer and colorectal adenocarcinoma. Furthermore, the different value that p53 and angiogenesis seem to have in predicting response to therapy and prognosis in locally advanced head and neck and ovarian cancers is of potential clinical relevance and needs to be confirmed by other authors and in larger series.

p53 and angiogenesis - different pathways leading to survival from hypoxia?

The reported differences in prediction of response to therapeutic modalities and survival may be related to recent observations regarding the role of p53 and survival under hypoxia. Cells that develop mutations in p53 may have a survival advantage, even without induction of angiogenesis [39]. There are therefore two different pathways by which tumours may enlarge in the presence of hypoxia-induced angiogenesis or reduce hypoxia-induced apoptosis. These pathways may be separately regulated and, indeed, this appears to be the case for many tumours, with no association of p53 with angiogenesis. However, in this case

one would expect both pathways to produce independent information on survival.

When treatment is given the situation is more complicated. Although one
would expect high angiogenesis to be associated with good oxygenation and
good response to radiation therapy, in actual fact antiangiogenic drugs potenti-
ate radiation therapy [40] and this may be because highly vascular tumours
may also have shunts and poorly perfused areas. Thus, in head and neck cancer
high angiogenesis was associated with poor response to radiation [29]. In contrast, for drugs with a greater diffusion, oxygen vascularisation may be related
to response.

The role of p53 is more complex because of the associated genetic instability
and anti-apoptotic role. Even with good initial responses to therapy, cells may
undergo further genetic changes resulting in poor survival. The clinical and laboratory studies mentioned above suggest that the combined blockade of both
pathways may be a highly synergistic therapeutic strategy [41,42].

p53 and angiogenesis as targets for novel anticancer therapeutic strategies

p53 alteration and aberrant angiogenesis are two relevant pathways of tumour
progression; furthermore, it is possible to restore wtp53 and to inhibit angiogenesis by gene therapy or pharmacological interventions [41,42]. Therefore, it
seems reasonable to assume that the assessment of both these biological phenomena by the determination of adequate surrogate markers in the tumour tissue, may be predictive of response to modulation of p53 or angiogenesis in human
cancers [41,42]. Indeed, surrogate markers of p53 functions and angiogenesis
should be valid tools to identify, prior to therapy, those patients with tumours
which are more likely to respond to restoration of wtp53 and/or to angiogenesis
inhibitors.

An answer to the question whether or not p53 protein and microvessel density
or the expression of angiogenic peptides and endogenous angiogenesis inhibitors
are valid surrogate markers to predict the efficacy of the respective biological
treatments, will require extensive translational research during the years to
come.

Future directions of research

Owing to recent developments in DNA sequencing technology it will soon be possible to sequence the p53 gene in individual patients at a cost similar to that of
receptor immunohistochemical analysis. Similarly, improved imaging techniques such as positron emission tomography or use of labelled antibodies specific for tumour endothelium will allow assessment of blood flow and vascula-
ture *in vivo*.

As new treatments to inhibit both pathways are developed, the diagnostic
ability is likely to improve and needs to be incorporated into treatment plan-
ning.

Acknowledgement

This work was supported in part by grants from the "Associazione Italiana per la Ricerca sul Cancro" (A.I.R.C.), Milan, Italy.

References

1   Chang F, Syrjanen S, Syrjanen K. Implications of p53 tumor suppressor gene in clinical oncology (review). J Clin Oncol 1995; 13: 1009-22
2   Marx J. Learning how to suppress cancer. Science 1993; 261: 1385-7
3   Bouck N. p53 and angiogenesis. Biochem Biophys Acta 1996; 1287: 63-6
4   Dameron KM, Volpert OV, Tainsky MA, Bouck N. Control of angiogenesis in fibroblasts by p53 regulation of thrombospondin-1. Science 1994; 265: 1582-5
5   Stellmach V, Volpert OV, Crawford SE, Lawler J, Hynes RO, Bouck N. Tumor suppressor genes and angiogenesis: the role of TP53 in fibroblasts. Eur J Cancer 1996; 32A: 2394-400
6   Volpert OV, Stellmach V, Bouck N. The modulation of thrombospondin and other naturally occurring inhibitors of angiogenesis during tumor progression. Breast Cancer Res Treat 1995; 36: 119-26
7   Van Meier EG, Polverini PJ, Chazin VR, Su Huang H-J, de Tribolet N, Cavanee WK. Release of an inhibitor of angiogenesis upon induction of wild-type p53 expression in glioblastoma cells. Nature Genetics 1994; 8: 171-6
8   Mulkhopadhway D, Tsiokas L, Sukhatame VP. Wild-type p53 and v-src exert opposing influences on human vascular endothelial growth factor gene expression. Cancer Res 1995; 55: 6161-5
9   Kieser A, Wiech HA, Brandner G, Marmé D, Kolch W. Mutant p53 potentiates protein kinase C induction of vascular endothelial growth factor expression. Oncogene 1994; 9: 963-9
10   Dietrich C, Bartsch T, Schanz F, Oesch F, Wieser RJ. p53-dependent cell cycle arrest induced by N-acetyl-L-leucinyl-L-leucinyl-L-norleucinal in platelet-derived growth factor-stimulated human fibroblasts. Proc Natl Acad Sci USA 1996; 93: 10815-9
11   Stromblad S, Cheresh DA. Cell adhesion and angiogenesis. Trends Cell Biol 1996; 6: 462-8
12   Brooks PC, Clark RAF, Cheresh DA. Requirement of vascular $\alpha_v\beta_3$ for angiogenesis. Science 1994; 264: 569-71
13   Friedlander M, Brooks PC, Shaffer RW, Kincaid CM, Varner JA, Cheresh DA. Definition of 2 angiogenic pathways by distinct α_v integrins. Science 1995; 270: 1500-2
14   Brooks PC, Montgomery AMP, Rosenfeld M et al. Integrin $\alpha_v\beta_3$ antagonists promote tumor regression by inducing apoptosis of angiogenic blood vessels. Cell 1994; 79: 1157-64
15   Stromblad S, Becker JC, Yebra M, Brooks PC, Cheresh DA. Suppression of p53 activity and p21$^{WAF1/CIP1}$ expression by vascular cell integrin $\alpha_v\beta_3$ during angiogenesis. J Clin Invest 1996; 98: 426-33
16   Bates S, Vousden KH. p53 in signaling checkpoint arrest or apoptosis. Curr Opin Genet Devel 1996; 6: 12-8
17   Gasparini G. p53 and angiogenesis (letter). J Clin Oncol 1995; 13: 1830
18   Horak ER, Leek R, Klenk N et al. Angiogenesis, assessed by platelet/endothelial cell adhesion molecule antibodies, as indicator of node metastases and survival in breast cancer. Lancet 1992; 340: 1120-4
19   Toi M, Kashitani J, Tominaga T. Tumor angiogenesis is an independent prognostic indicator in primary breast carcinoma. Int J Cancer 1993; 55: 371-4

20 Gasparini G, Bevilacqua P, Boracchi P et al. Prognostic value of p53 expression in early-stage breast carcinoma compared with tumour angiogenesis, epidermal growth factor receptor, c-erbB-2, cathepsin D, DNA ploidy, parameters of cell kinetics and conventional features. Int J Oncol 1994; 4: 155-62

21 Gasparini G, Weidner N, Bevilacqua P et al. Tumor microvessel density, p53 expression, tumor size and peritumoral lymphatic vessel invasion are relevant prognostic markers in node-negative breast carcinoma. J Clin Oncol 1994; 12: 454-66

22 Bevilacqua P, Barbareschi M, Verderio P et al. Prognostic value of intratumoral microvessel density, a measure of tumor angiogenesis, in node-negative breast carcinoma. Results of a multiparametric study. Breast Cancer Res Treat 1995; 36: 205-17

23 Costello P, McCann A, Carney DN, Dervan PA. Prognostic significance of microvessel density in lymph node negative breast carcinoma. Hum Pathol 1995; 26: 1181-4

24 Gasparini G, Toi M, Verderio P et al. Prognostic significance of p53, angiogenesis, and other conventional features in operable breast cancer. Subanalysis in node-positive and node-negative patients. J Exp Ther Oncol 1997; 2: 1-9

25 Weidner N, Semple JP, Welch WR, Folkman J. Tumor angiogenesis and metastasis - correlation in invasive breast carcinoma. N Engl J Med 1991; 324: 1-8

26 Vermeulen PB, Gasparini G, Fox SB et al. Quantification of angiogenesis in solid human tumours: An international consensus on the methodology and criteria of evaluation. Eur J Cancer 1996; 32A: 2474-84

27 Elledge RM. Assessing p53 status in breast cancer prognosis: Where should you put the thermometer if you think your p53 is sick? J Natl Cancer Inst 1996; 98: 141-3

28 Gasparini G, Weidner N, Maluta S et al. Intratumoral microvessel density and p53 protein: correlation with metastasis in head and neck squamous-cell carcinoma. Int J Cancer 1993; 55: 739-44

29 Gasparini G, Bevilacqua P, Bonoldi E et al. Predictive and prognostic markers in a series of patients with head and neck squamous-cell invasive carcinoma treated with concurrent chemoradiation therapy. Clin Cancer Res 1995; 1: 1375-83

30 Gasparini G, Bonoldi E, Viale G et al. Prognostic and predictive value of tumour angiogenesis in ovarian carcinomas. Int J Cancer 1996; 69: 205-11

31 Bochner BH, Nichols PW, Esrig D et al. Relationship between p53 and tumour angiogenesis in invasive transitional cell carcinoma (TCC) of the bladder. Proc Am Assoc Cancer Res 1995; 36: 91 (abstr 541)

32 Bochner BH, Cote RJ, Weidner N et al. Angiogenesis in bladder cancer: Relationship between microvessel density and tumor prognosis. J Natl Cancer Inst 1995; 87: 1603-12

33 Grossfeld GD, Ginsberg DA, Stein JP et al. Thrombospondin-1 expression in bladder cancer: association with p53 alterations, tumor angiogenesis and tumor progression. J Natl Cancer Inst 1997; 89: 219-27

34 O'Brien TS, Fox SB, Dickinson AJ et al. Expression of the angiogenic factor thymidine phosphorylase/platelet-derived endothelial cell growth factor in primary bladder cancers. Cancer Res 1996; 56: 4799-804

35 Giatromanolaki A, Koukourakis M, O'Byrne K et al. Prognostic value of angiogenesis in operable non-small cell lung cancer. J Pathol 1996; 179: 80-8

36 Fontanini G, Vignati S, Lucchi M et al. Neoangiogenesis and p53 protein in lung cancer: their prognostic role and their relationship with vascular endothelial growth factor (VEGF) expression. Br J Cancer 1997; in press

37 Vermeulen PB, Roland L, Martens V et al. Correlation of intratumoral microvessel density and p53 protein overexpression in human colorectal adenocarcinoma. Microvasc Res 1996; 51: 164-74

38 Pezzella F, Di Bacco A, Andreola S, Nicholson AG, Pastorino U, Harris AL. Angiogenesis in primary lung cancer and lung secondaries. Eur J Cancer 1996; 32A: 2494-500

39 Graeber TG, Osmanian C, Jacks T et al. Hypoxia-mediated selection of cells with diminished apoptotic potential in solid tumours. Nature 1996; 379: 88-91

40 Teicher BA, Holden SA, Dupuis NP et al. Potentiation of cytotoxic therapies by TNP-470 and minocycline in mice bearing EMT-6 mammary carcinoma. Breast Cancer Res Treat 1995; 36: 227-36
41 Harris CC. Structure and function of the p53 tumor suppressor gene: Clues for rational cancer therapeutic strategies (review). J Natl Cancer Inst 1996; 88: 1442-5
42 Gasparini G. Antiangiogenic drugs as a novel anticancer therapeutic strategy. Which are the more promising agents? Which are the clinical developments and indications? (review). Critical Rev Oncol/Hematol 1997; in press

ESO Scientific Updates, Vol. 1
Prognostic and Predictive Value of p53
J.G.M. Klijn, editor
© 1997 Elsevier Science B.V. All rights reserved

Prognostic and Predictive Value of p53 Aberrations in Tumours of the Gastrointestinal Tract and Pancreas

Giuseppe Viale

Department of Pathology and Laboratory Medicine, European Institute of Oncology, University of Milan School of Medicine, Milan, Italy

Introduction

p53 aberrations, either in the form of mutations of the gene and/or accumulation of the encoded protein, have been quite extensively investigated in tumours of the gastrointestinal tract. The studies have consistently documented the occurrence of p53 aberrations in a high percentage of oesophageal, gastric and colorectal carcinomas, as well as in some preneoplastic conditions, such as Barrett's oesophagus and gastric dysplasia. p53 mutations have also been implicated as a late event in the adenoma-carcinoma sequence of colorectal cancer.

The prognostic and predictive implications of p53 aberrations in these tumours, however, are much more debated. Indeed, in a similar manner as for malignancies of other organs, different investigations aimed at evaluating the prognostic and predictive role of p53 mutations and/or accumulation in gastrointestinal carcinomas have provided contrasting results. The reasons for these discrepancies may be manyfold, and include the evaluation of series of cases with variable numbers of patients and different length of follow-up, the use of different methodological approaches (immunocytochemistry, SSCP analysis, sequencing) to the assessment of p53 aberrations, the use of diverse statistical analyses for the evaluation of the results, with multivariate analyses having been performed in a minority of the studies.

Because immunocytochemistry has been most commonly used for analysing p53 status, the variables of the staining protocols and of the scoring systems may be responsible for most of the discrepant findings. In fact, different polyclonal and monoclonal antibodies to p53 have been used in these studies, and different pretreatments of the tissue sections before immunostaining have been

---

Address for correspondence: G. Viale, Department of Pathology and Laboratory Medicine, European Institute of Oncology, Via Ripamonti 435, 20141 Milano, Italy. Tel.: +39-2-57489419, Fax: +39-2-57489417, e-mail: gviale@ieo.cilea.it

performed. Furthermore, the methods used for evaluating the immunostaining results are disappointingly variable, with some authors regarding positive cases irrespective of the percentage of the neoplastic cells showing immunoreactivity, whereas others require staining of a variable percentage (from 5% to 50%) of neoplastic cells for a case to be considered positive. Also, the subcellular compartmentalisation of the immunoreactivity (i.e., nuclear vs cytoplasmic staining) has been variably considered, with some investigators disregarding cytoplasmic immunoreactivity as non-specific, whereas others have taken it into account.

A minority of investigations have used molecular biology techniques for assessing the prognostic value of p53 gene abnormalities in gastrointestinal cancers. Most of these studies, however, did not include sequencing of the gene, and therefore they did not provide any data on the possible different biological and clinical implications of specific mutations.

Oesophageal cancer

p53 gene mutations have been detected in 42% to 67% of oesophageal carcinomas [1-4], with only two studies reporting a much lower (8%) [5] or much higher (84%) [6] prevalence. Nuclear p53 protein accumulation has been identified in a more variable percentage of cases (from 34% to 87%) [3,7-11], irrespective of the histological type of the neoplasms (squamous cell carcinomas or adenocarcinomas). When both immunocytochemical and molecular biology techniques were used for analysing the same tumours, however, discordant results were obtained in 24% to 45% of the cases [2,3,10].

The appearance of p53 aberrations is likely to represent an early event in oesophageal carcinogenesis. Indeed, nuclear accumulation of p53 protein has been documented in low- and high-grade oesophageal dysplasia coexisting with squamous cell carcinoma [12,13] and in Barrett's oesophagus as well [14-16]. In this latter condition, the prevalence of p53 accumulation correlates with increasing grades of dysplasia [15,16]. Furthermore, an identical mutation of the p53 gene was identified in a biopsy specimen showing a high-grade dysplastic area and in the intramucosal carcinoma developed at the same site one year later [17].

The prognostic value of p53 aberrations in oesophageal carcinomas is much more controversial. Preliminary investigations reported a significantly shorter overall survival for patients carrying oesophageal squamous cell carcinomas with nuclear p53 accumulation [8,18,19]. These investigations, however, could not document any independent prognostic value of p53 accumulation because multivariate analyses of the results were not performed. Sarbia and coworkers [20] and Duhaylongsod and coworkers [9], however, were unable to find any association between p53 accumulation and patient survival either in squamous cell carcinomas or in adenocarcinomas. In one series [21] p53 accumulation was correlated with improved survival of patients with oesophageal adenocarcinoma. We have examined p53 accumulation and mutations in a series of 74 patients, using both immunocytochemistry and PCR-SSCP analysis of exons 5 to 8 of the p53 gene [22]. Overall, 54 (73%) cases displayed p53 accumulation and/or mutations, but p53 aberrations were not correlated with patient survival.

Gastric carcinoma

The reported prevalence of p53 accumulation in gastric carcinomas ranges between 23% [23] and 70% [24], while p53 mutations have been detected in 28% [23] to 50% [25] of the cases. Most studies indicated a higher prevalence of p53 aberrations in intestinal-type adenocarcinomas than in diffuse carcinomas, but this correlation has not been confirmed in others [26].

Just as for oesophageal carcinomas, p53 aberrations are likely to represent an early event in gastric carcinogenesis (at least for the intestinal-type adenocarcinomas), because they are already detectable in dysplastic lesions [24,27,28].

Nuclear p53 accumulation has been reported in more than 60% of intestinal-type adenomas [29], and the extent of immunoreactivity was significantly greater in cases showing high-grade epithelial dysplasia. Conversely, p53 accumulation was found in only 3 of 18 gastric-type adenomas, all displaying high-grade epithelial dysplasia. Similar findings were reported by Imatami et al. [30], who detected p53 accumulation in 7 of 39 adenomas, but in none of 33 cases of regenerative atypia.

In the incomplete type of intestinal metaplasia p53 accumulation [27,30-32] and mutations [27,31,32] are already detectable, thus reinforcing the hypothesis that this type of metaplasia may contain precursor lesions of gastric adenocarcinoma.

The possible prognostic implications of p53 aberrations in gastric carcinomas remain controversial. Indeed, two studies [26,33] reported a significant association of p53 accumulation with a worse survival, which was independent of other factors in multivariate analysis. This association, however, was not confirmed by other investigations [23,34-37] which failed to document any independent prognostic role of p53 accumulation in gastric carcinomas. Interestingly, one study [23] included analysis of the p53 gene (exons 5-8) by PCR-SSCP and documented p53 mutations in 28% of the cases. In multivariate analysis, p53 mutations (but not nuclear p53 accumulation) correlated independently with poor survival.

Finally, two studies recently reported an association of nuclear accumulation of p53 with a poor response to chemotherapy and radiotherapy [38,39].

Colorectal carcinoma

Colorectal carcinomas have been extensively studied for p53 aberrations. The reported prevalence of nuclear p53 accumulation in these tumours ranges from

42% [40] to 69% [41]. p53 gene abnormalities have been detected in 52% [42] to 80% [43] of the cases investigated.

p53 aberrations most likely play a crucial role as a late event in the transition from adenoma to carcinoma. Indeed, the vast majority of colorectal adenomas with mild and moderate dysplasia do not show any p53 accumulation [44,45] or p53 gene mutation [46], whereas adenomas with severe dysplasia exhibit nuclear accumulation of p53 protein [45,47] to the same extent as colorectal adenocarcinomas.

Also, p53 accumulation has been detected in dysplastic epithelia of ulcerative colitis patients, and correlated positively with increasing grades of dysplasia [43].

At least 30 investigations have dealt with the prognostic significance of p53 aberrations in colorectal adenocarcinomas (Table 1). In the vast majority of these studies immunocytochemistry was used to document an abnormal accumulation of p53 protein in the neoplastic cells. As anticipated in the introduction to this chapter, the variables related to the immunocytochemical methods for p53 accumulation are so numerous that it is almost impossible to compare the results of different studies. However, of the 25 investigations using immunocytochemistry, 10 documented a significant inverse correlation of p53 accumulation with patient survival, whereas 15 did not. Similarly, 2 of the 5 investigations assessing the status of the p53 gene reported a significant inverse correlation of p53 gene abnormalities with patient survival, whereas the remaining 3 failed to find such a correlation.

Despite the great discrepancy in the findings and conclusions reported thus far, some intriguing and interesting data emerge from the literature. We and others [49,53,67] have documented that cytoplasmic p53 accumulation (after immunostaining with the CM1 polyclonal antiserum) is an independent predictor of reduced survival, especially for patients with tumours of the left colon and rectum, whereas nuclear accumulation is not. The cytoplasmic accumulation of p53 protein in our series was correlated with the lack of mutations in exons 5 to 8, whereas nuclear p53 accumulation was correlated with the occurrence of mutations in these conserved exons [59]. Interestingly, Leahy et al. [70] also investigated a series of 66 cases both with immunocytochemistry (DO-7 monoclonal antibody) and PCR-SSCP analysis of exons 5 to 8, and found that SSCP abnormalities were unrelated to the immunocytochemical expression of p53. When they analysed survival of the patients with multivariate analysis, p53 overexpression emerged as an independent prognostic variable, whereas SSCP abnormalities did not.

It can be deduced from the above data that nuclear and/or cytoplasmic p53 accumulation is likely to have some prognostic implications in colorectal adenocarcinomas, although it does not reflect mutations in the highly conserved domains of the p53 gene. Alternative mechanisms of p53 inactivation and accumulation should therefore be active in these tumours, and be correlated with a more aggressive clinical course.

Table 1. Prognostic significance of p53 aberrations in colorectal carcinomas

First author	Method	No. positive (%)	Follow-up	p value
Scott [40]	IHC	72/125 (42%)	35 months	N.S.
Remvikos [48]	FCM	52/78 (67%)	42 months	0.03
Sun [49]	IHC	73/293 (25%)	>5 yrs	<0.001
Starzynska [50]	IHC	49/107 (46%)	12 months	0.001
Yamaguchi [51]	IHC	61/100 (61%)	6-48 months	0.05
Bell [52]	IHC	45/100 (45%)	34 months	N.S.
Bosari [53]	IHC	99/197 (50%)	>5 yrs	0.0017
Hamelin [42]	DGGE	44/85 (52%)	47 months	0.003
Auvinen [41]	IHC	100/144 (69%)	>9 yrs	N.S.
Nathanson [54]	IHC	52/84 (62%)	>5 yrs	N.S.
Tanaka [55]	IHC	23/36 (64%)	>2 yrs	N.A.
Zeng [56]	IHC	50/107 (47%)	62 months	0.02 (DFS)
Morrin [57]	IHC	32/52 (62%)	>5 yrs	N.S.
Mulder [58]	IHC	43/109 (40%)	>7 yrs	N.S.
Bosari [59]	SSCP	74/126	>5 yrs	N.S.
Diez [60]	IHC	27/61 (44%)	46 months	0.012 (DFS)
Ofner [61]	IHC	60/109 (55%)	79 months	N.S.
Grewal [62]	IHC	34/66 (51.5%)	45 months	N.S.
Lazaris [63]	IHC	28/60 (46.6%)	>5 yrs	<0.01
Kressner [64]	IHC	162/294 (55%)	4.5 yrs	N.S.
Pricolo [65]	SEQ	43/70 (61%)	5 yrs	0.006 (sg III)
Lanza [66]	IHC	124/204 (61%)	33 months	N.S.
Flamini [67]	IHC	45/96 (47%)	36 m	0.002 (N.S.)
Baretton [68]	IHC	60/101 (59%)	8 yrs	0.009
Slebos [69]	IHC	21/46 (46%)	N.A.	N.S.
	SEQ	19/46 (41%)		N.S.
Lanza [66]	IHC	124/204 (61%)	33.4 months	N.S.
Leahy [70]	IHC	34/66 (52%)	9.9 yrs	0.001
	SSCP	27/66 (41%)		N.S.
Poller [71]	IHC	152/250 (61%)	4.3 yrs	N.S.

IHC = immunohistochemistry; FCM = flow cytometry; DGGE = denaturing gel gradient electrophoresis; SSCP = single strand conformation polymorphism; SEQ = sequencing; N.A. = not available; N.S. = not significant; DFS = disease-free survival; sgIII = stage III

More recently, emphasis has also been placed on the expression of p21 (CIP1), an inhibitor of cyclin/cyclin-dependent kinases. p21 is induced by wild-type p53 and blocks the G1/S transition of the cell cycle. Down-regulated expression of p21 has already been documented in colorectal carcinomas [69,72], though the relationships between p21 immunoreactivity and p53 accumulation or mutations are still to be elucidated. Indeed, Slebos et al. [69] did not find any correlation between p21 staining and p53 aberrations, whereas Matsushita et al. [72] reported that the relative mRNA expression of p21 was lower in tumours with p53 mutations than in those without.

We have found a strong inverse correlation between p21 immunoreactivity, p53 nuclear accumulation (p=0.007) and p53 mutations in exons 5 to 8 (p=0.0007) in a series of 200 colorectal carcinomas. p21 immunoreactivity was also inversely correlated with the stage of the tumours. As a consequence, in multivariate analysis of survival immunoreactivity for p21 did not show any independent prognostic value [73].

Pancreatic adenocarcinoma

p53 accumulation and mutations are as common in pancreatic adenocarcinomas as in tumours of the gastrointestinal tract, ranging from 40% [74,75] to 60% [76] of the cases. It has been suggested that an altered p53 gene might cooperate with activated Ki-ras in the malignant transformation of the pancreatic ductal epithelium [77].

Overexpression of p53 has also been documented in *in situ* carcinomas and in hyperplastic lesions with and without dysplasia, thus suggesting that p53 abnormalities are an early event in the development of pancreatic adenocarcinomas [75].

Comparatively few investigations have dealt with the prognostic significance of p53 aberrations in these malignancies. Nuclear p53 accumulation has been reported as an independent prognostic parameter by Yokoyama et al. [78] and Aizawa et al. [79], but other groups failed to document any prognostic significance of p53 accumulation [74,80]. One single study reported an adverse effect of p53 mutations (detected in 29 of 71 cases) on patient survival [81].

Epilogue

In the 17 years following the discovery of the p53 tumour suppressor gene, great effort has been made to assess its actual role in neoplastic transformation and tumour progression. More recently, emphasis has been placed also on the implications of p53 for the susceptibility of tumours to different therapeutic regimens, and on the possibility of targeting it for genetic interventions.

Crucial for most of these issues is the assessment of the actual predictive and prognostic value of this gene in human malignancies. Unfortunately, despite the very large amount of research into the subject, the possible clinical consequences of p53 aberrations are still incompletely established.

There is a need for standardisation of the technical approach to assess p53 aberrations, large series of cases with adequate follow-up should be studied, and multivariate analyses of the results should be consistently performed.

Multicentre studies with centralised testing facilities could be of great value in providing definitive answers to the many questions that are still open.

Acknowledgement

The skillful editorial assistance of Dr Mariachiara Novati is gratefully acknowledged.

References

1   Hollstein MC, Peri L, Mandard AM et al. Genetic analysis of human oesophageal tumors from two high incidence geographic areas: frequent p53 base substitutions and absence of ras mutations. Cancer Res 1991; 51: 4102-6

2   Gao H, Wang L-D, Zhou Q, Hong J-Y, Huang T-Y, Yang CS. p53 tumor suppressor gene mutation in early esophageal precancerous lesions and carcinoma among high-risk populations in Henan, China. Cancer Res 1994; 54: 4342-6

3   Wagata T, Shibagaki I, Imamura M et al. Loss of 17p, mutations of the p53 gene, and overexpression of p53 protein in esophageal squamous cell carcinomas. Cancer Res 1993; 53: 846-50

4   Neshat K, Sanchez CA, Galipeau PC et al. p53 mutations in Barrett's adenocarcinoma and high grade dysplasia. Gastroenterology 1994; 106: 1589-95

5   Casson AG, Mukhopadhyay T, Cleary KR, Ro JY, Levin B, Roth J. p53 gene mutations in Barrett's epithelium and esophageal cancer. Cancer Res 1991; 51: 4495-9

6   Audrezet MP, Robaszkiewicz M, Mercier B et al. TP53 gene mutation profile in esophageal squamous cell carcinomas. Cancer Res 1993; 53: 5745-9

7   Younes M, Lebovitz RM, Lechago LV, Lechago J. p53 protein accumulation in Barrett's metaplasia, dysplasia and carcinoma: a follow-up study. Gastroenterology 1993; 105: 1637-42

8   Shimaya K, Shiozaki H, Inoue M, Tahara H, Monden T, Shimano T, Mori T. Significance of p53 expression as a prognostic factor in oesophageal squamous cell carcinoma. Virchows Archiv A Pathol Anat Histopathol 1993; 422: 271-6

9   Duhaylongsod FG, Gottfried MR, Iglehart JD, Vaughn AL, Wolfe WG. The significance of c-erb B-2 and p53 immunoreactivity in patients with adenocarcinoma of the esophagus. Ann Surg 1995; 221: 677-84

10 Moore JH, Lesser EJ, Erdody DH, Natale RB, Orringer MB, Beer DG. Intestinal differentiation and p53 gene alterations in Barrett's esophagus and esophageal adenocarcinoma. Int J Cancer 1994; 56: 487-93

11 Jaskiewicz K, De Groot KM. p53 gene mutants expression, cellular proliferation and differentiation in oesophageal carcinoma and non-cancerous epithelium. Anticancer Res 1994; 14: 137-40

12 Parenti AR, Rugge M, Frizzera E et al. p53 overexpression in the multistep process of oesophageal carcinogenesis. Am J Surg Pathol 1995; 19: 1418-22

13 Itakura Y, Sasano F, Date F et al. DNA ploidy, p53 expression, and cellular proliferation in normal epithelium and squamous dysplasia of non-cancerous and cancerous human oesophagi. Anticancer Res 1996; 16: 201-8

14 Symmans PJ, Linehan JM, Brito MJ, Filipe MI. p53 expression in Barrett's oesophagus, dysplasia, and adenocarcinoma using antibody DO-7. J Pathol 1995; 173: 221-6

15 Polkowski W, van Lanschot JJ, Ten Kate FJ et al. The value of p53 and Ki67 as markers for tumour progression in the Barrett's dysplasia-carcinoma sequence. Surg Oncol 1995; 4: 163-71

16 Flejou JF, Diebold MD, Sagan C et al. Overexpression of protein p53 and Barrett esophagus. A frequent and early event in the course of carcinogenesis. Gastroenterol Clin Biol 1995; 19: 475-81

17 Audrezet MP, Robaszkiewicz M, Mercier B et al. Molecular analysis of the TP53 gene in Barrett's adenocarcinoma. Hum Mutat 1996; 7: 109-13

18 Furihata M, Ohtsuki Y, Takahashi A, Tamiya T, Ogata T. Prognostic significance of human papillomavirus genome (type-16, -18) and aberrant expression of p53 protein in human esophageal cancer. Int J Cancer 1993; 54: 220-30

19 Wang D-Y, Xiang Y-Y, Tanaka M, Li X-R, Li J-L, Shen Q, Sugimura H, Kino I. High prevalence of p53 protein overexpression in patients with esophageal cancer in Linxian, China and its relationship to progression and prognosis. Cancer 1994; 74: 3089-96

20 Sarbia M, Porschen R, Borchard F, Horstmann O, Willers R, Gabbert HE. p53 protein expression and prognosis in squamous cell carcinoma of the esophagus. Cancer 1994; 74: 2218-23

21 Sauter ER, Keller SM, Erner SM. p53 correlates with improved survival in patients with esophageal adenocarcinoma. J Surg Oncol 1995; 58: 269-73

22 Coggi G, Bosari S, Roncalli M et al. p53 protein accumulation and p53 gene mutation in esophageal cancer: a molecular and immunohistochemical study with clinicopathological correlations. Cancer 1997; 79: 425-32

23 Lim BHG, Soong R, Grieu F, Robbins PD, House AK, Iacopetta BJ. p53 accumulation and mutation are prognostic indicators of poor survival in human gastric carcinoma. Int J Cancer 1996; 69: 200-4

24 Craanen ME, Blok P, Dekker W, Offerhaus GJ, Tytgat GN. Chronology of p53 protein accumulation in gastric carcinogenesis. Gut 1995; 36: 848-52

25 Ranzani GN, Luinetti O, Padovan LS et al. p53 gene mutations and protein nuclear accumulation are early events in intestinal type gastric cancer but late events in diffuse type. Cancer Epidemiol Biomarkers Prev 1995; 4: 223-31

26 Joypaul BV, Hopwood D, Newman EL. The prognostic significance of the accumulation of p53 tumour-suppressor gene protein in gastric adenocarcinoma. Br J Cancer 1994; 69: 943-6

27 Shiao Y-H, Rugge M, Correa P, Lehmann HP, Scheer WD. p53 alteration in gastric precancerous lesions. Am J Pathol 1994; 144: 511-7

28 Miracco C, Spina D, Vindigni C, Filipe MI, Tosi P. Cell proliferation patterns and p53 expression in gastric dysplasia. Int J Cancer 1995; 62: 149-54

29 Kushima R, Muller W, Stolte M, Borchard F. Differential p53 protein expression in stomach adenomas of gastric and intestinal phenotypes: possible sequences of p53 alteration in stomach carcinogenesis. Virchows Arch 1996; 428: 223-7

30 Imatani A, Sasano H, Asaki S et al. Analysis of p53 abnormalities in endoscopic gastric biopsies. Anticancer Res 1996; 16: 2049-56

31 Gomyo Y, Osaki M, Kaibara N, Ito H. Numerical aberration and point mutation of p53 gene in human gastric intestinal metaplasia and well-differentiated adenocarcinoma: analysis by fluorescence in situ hybridization (FISH) and PCR-SSCP. Int J Cancer 1996; 66: 594-9

32 Ochiai A, Yamauchi Y, Hirohashi S. p53 mutations in non-neoplastic mucosa of the human stomach showing intestinal metaplasia. Int J Cancer 1996; 69: 28-33

33 Martin HM, Filipe MI, Morris RW, Lane DP, Sivestre F. p53 expression and prognosis in gastric carcinoma. Int J Cancer 1992; 50: 859-62

34 Kakeji Y, Korenaga D, Tsujitani S et al. Gastric cancer with p53 overexpression has high potential for metastasising to lymph nodes. Br J Cancer 1993; 67: 589-93

35 Hurlimann J. Prognostic value of p53 protein expression in breast carcinomas. Path Res Pract 1993; 189: 996-1003

36 Gabbert HE, Muller W, Schneiders A, Meier S, Hommel G. The relationship of p53 expression to the prognosis of 418 patients with gastric carcinoma. Cancer 1995; 76: 720-6

37 Victorzon M, Nordling S, Haglund C, Lundin J, Roberts PJ. Expression of p53 protein as a prognostic factor in patients with gastric cancer. Eur J Cancer 1996; 32A: 215-20

38 Nakata B, Chung YS, Ogawa M et al. Association between p53 expression and chemosensitivity in advanced and recurrent gastric cancer. Gan To Kagaku Ryoho 1996; 23: 151-3

39 Hamada M, Fujiwara T, Hizuta A et al. The p53 gene is a potent determinant of chemosensitivity and radiosensitivity in gastric and colorectal cancers. J Cancer Res Clin Oncol 1996; 122: 360-5

40 Scott NP, Sagar P, Stewart J, Blair GE, Dixon MF, Quirke P. p53 in colorectal cancer: clinicopathological correlations and prognostic significance. Br J Cancer 1991; 63: 317-9

41 Auvinen A, Isola J, Visakorpi T, Koivula T, Virtanen S, Hakama M. Overexpression of p53 and long-term survival in colon carcinoma. Br J Cancer 1994; 70: 293-6

42 Hamelin R, Laurent-Puig P, Olshwang S et al. Association of p53 mutations with short survival in colorectal cancer. Gastroenterology 1994; 106: 42-8

43 Harpaz N, Peck AL, Yin J et al. p53 protein expression in ulcerative colitis-associated colorectal dysplasia and carcinoma. Hum Pathol 1994; 25: 1069-74

44 Purdie CA, O'Grady J, Piris J, Wyllie AH, Bird CC. p53 expression in colorectal tumors. Am J Pathol 1991; 138: 807-13

45 Sameshima S, Kubota Y, Sawada T et al. Overexpression of p53 protein and histologic grades of dysplasia in colorectal adenomas. Dis Colon Rectum 1996; 39: 562-7

46 Tominaga O, Hameli R, Trouvat V et al. Frequently elevated content of immuno-chemically defined wild-type p53 protein in colorectal adenomas. Oncogene 1993; 8: 2653-8

47 Ieda S, Watatani M, Yoshida T, Kuroda K, Inui H, Yasutomi M. Immunohistochemical analysis of p53 and ras p21 expression in colorectal adenomas and early carcinomas. Surg Today 1996; 26: 230-5

48 Remvikos Y, Tominaga O, Hammel P et al. Increased p53 protein content of colorectal tumors correlates with poor survival. Br J Cancer 1992; 66: 758-64

49 Sun X-F, Carstensen JM, Zhang H et al. Prognostic significance of cytoplasmic p53 oncoprotein in colorectal adenocarcinoma. Lancet 1992; 340: 1369-73

50 Starzynska T, Bromley M, Ghohsh A, Stern PL. Prognostic significance of p53 over-expression in gastric and colorectal cancer. Br J Cancer 1992; 66: 558-62

51 Yamaguchi A, Kurosaka Y, Fushida S et al. Expression of p53 protein in colorectal cancer and it relationship to short-term prognosis. Cancer 1992; 70: 2778-84

52 Bell SM, Scott N, Cross D et al. Prognostic value of p53 overexpression and c-Ki-ras mutations in colorectal cancer. Gastroenterology 1993; 104: 57-64

53 Bosari S, Viale G, Bossi P et al. Cytoplasmic accumulation of p53 protein: an independent prognostic indicator in colorectal adenocarcinomas. J Natl Cancer Inst 1994; 86: 681-7

54 Nathanson SD, Linden MD, Tender P, Zarbo RJ, Jacobsen G, Nelson LT. Relationship among p53, stage, and prognosis of large bowel cancer. Dis Colon Rectum 1994; 37: 527-34

55 Tanaka M, Omura K, Watanabe Y, Oda Y, Nakanishi I. Prognostic factors of colorectal cancer: K-ras mutation, overexpression of the p53 protein, and cell proliferative activity. J Surg Oncol 1994; 57: 57-64

56 Zeng Z-S, Sarkis AS, Zhang Z-F et al. p53 nuclear overexpression: an independent predictor of survival in lymph node-positive colorectal cancer patients. J Clin Oncol 1994; 12: 2043-50

57 Morrin M, Kelly M, Barrett N, Delaney P. Mutations of Ki-ras and p53 genes in colorectal cancer and their prognostic significance. Gut 1994; 35: 1627-31

58 Mulder J-WR, Baas IO, Polak MM, Goodman SN, Offerhaus GJA. Evaluation of p53 protein expression as a marker for long-term prognosis in colorectal carcinoma. Br J Cancer 1995; 71: 1257-62

59 Bosari S, Viale G, Roncalli M et al. p53 gene mutations, p53 protein accumulation and compartmentalization in colorectal adenocarcinoma. Am J Pathol 1995; 147: 790-8

60 Diez M, Enriquez JM, Camunas J et al. Prediction of recurrence in B-C stages of colorectal cancer by p53 nuclear overexpression in comparison with standard pathological features. Eur J Surg Oncol 1995; 21: 635-9

61 Ofner D, Maier H, Riedmann B et al. Immunohistochemically detectable p53 and mdm-2 oncoprotein expression in colorectal carcinoma: prognostic significance. J Clin Pathol Mol Pathol 1995; 48: M12-M16

62 Grewal H, Guillem JG, Klimstra DS, Cohen AM. p53 nuclear overexpression may not be an independent prognostic marker in early colorectal cancer. Dis Colon Rectum 1995; 38: 1176-81

63 Lazaris AC, Theodoropoulos GE, Anastassopoulos P, Nakopoulou L, Panoussopoulos D, Papadimitriou K. Prognostic significance of p53 and c-erbB-2 immunohistochemical evaluation in colorectal adenocarcinoma. Histol Histopathol 1995; 10: 661-8

64 Kressner U, Lindmark G, Gerdin B, Pahlman L, Grimelius B. Immunohistological p53 staining is of limited value in the staging and prognostic prediction of colorectal cancer. Anticancer Res 1996; 16: 951-7

65 Pricolo VE, Finkelstein SD, Wu T-T et al. Prognostic value of TP53 and K-ras-2 mutational analysis in stage III carcinoma of the colon. Am J Surg1996; 171: 41-6

66 Lanza G Jr, Maestri I, Dubini A et al. p53 expression in colorectal cancer: relation to tumor type, DNA ploidy pattern and short-term survival. Am J Clin Pathol 1996; 105: 604-12

67 Flamini G, Curigliano G, Ratto C et al. Prognostic significance of cytoplasmic p53 overexpression in colorectal cancer. An immunohistochemical analysis. Eur J Cancer 1996; 32A: 802-5

68 Baretton GB, Vogt M, Muller C et al. Prognostic significance of p53 expression, chromosome 17 copy number, and DNA ploidy in non-metastasized colorectal carcinomas (stages IB and II). Scand J Gastroenterol 1996; 31: 481-9

69 Slebos RCJ, Baas IO, Clement M et al. Clinical and pathological associations with p53 tumour-suppressor gene mutations and expression of p21WAF1/Cip1 in colorectal carcinoma. Br J Cancer 1996; 74: 165-71

70 Leahy DT, Salman R, Mulcahy H, Sheahan K, O'Donoghue DP, Parfrey NA. Prognostic significance of p53 abnormalities in colorectal carcinoma detected by PCR-SSCP and immunohistochemical analysis. J Pathol 1996; 180: 364-70

71 Poller DN, Baxter KJ, Shepherd NA. p53 and Rb1 protein expression: are they prognostically useful in colorectal cancer? Br J Cancer 1997; 75: 87-93

72 Matsushita K, Kobayashi S, Kato M et al. Reduced messenger RNA expression level of p21 CIP1 in human colorectal carcinoma tissues and its association with p53 gene mutation. Int J Cancer 1996; 69: 259-64

73 Viale G, Pellegrini C, Mazzarol G, Maisonneuve P, Silverman ML, Bosari S. p21 (WAF1/CIP1) expression correlates with disease stage and p53 mutations in colorectal cancer. Mod Pathol 1997; 10: 66A

74 DiGiuseppe JA, Hruban RH, Goodman SN et al. Overexpression of p53 protein in adenocarcinoma of the pancreas. Am J Clin Pathol 1994; 101: 684-8

75 Boschman CR, Stryker S, Reddy JK, Rao MS. Expression of p53 protein in precursor lesions and adenocarcinoma of human pancreas. Am J Pathol 1994; 145: 1291-5

76 Barton CM, Staddon SL, Hughes CM et al. Abnormalities of the p53 tumor suppressor gene in human pancreatic cancer. Br J Cancer 1991; 64: 1076-82

77 Wanebo HJ, Vezeridis MP. Pancreatic carcinoma in perspective. A continuing challenge. Cancer 1996; 78: 580-91

78 Yokoyama M, Yamanaka Y, Friess H, Buchler M, Korc M. p53 expression in human pancreatic cancer correlates with enhanced biological aggressiveness. Anticancer Res 1994; 14: 2477-83
79 Aizawa S, Sasaki M, Wada R, Koyama M, Yagihashi S. p53 protein expression in pancreatic tumors and its relationship to clinicopathological factors and prognosis. J Surg Oncol 1996; 62: 279-83
80 Lundin J, Nordling S, von Boguslawsky K, Roberts PJ, Haglund C. Prognostic value of immunohistochemical expression of p53 in patients with pancreatic cancer. Oncology 1996; 53: 104-11
81 Weyer K, Feichtinger H, Haun M et al. p53, Ki-ras, and DNA ploidy in human pancreatic ductal adenocarcinomas. Lab Invest 1996; 74: 279-89

ESO Scientific Updates, Vol. 1
Prognostic and Predictive Value of p53
J.G.M. Klijn, editor
© 1997 Elsevier Science B.V. All rights reserved

p53 Genotypes and Haplotypes with a Potentially Predictive Value for Risk Assessment and Retroviral p53 Transduction for Gene Therapy of Breast Cancer

Ingo B. Runnebaum

Department of Obstetrics and Gynaecology, Molecular Biology Laboratory, University of Ulm, Germany

Introduction

Susceptibility to breast cancer

Breast cancer is the most common cancer in women in Western countries. Susceptibility to breast cancer may be modified by the involvement of germ-line variations in genes that control cell proliferation, programmed cell death, repair of DNA damage, metabolism of carcinogens, production of endogenous carcinogens or defense mechanisms including immune response. One of the genes implicated in cancer development is the p53 gene involved in control of the cell cycle, apoptosis and DNA repair. Somatic mutations in the p53 gene have frequently been found in many different forms of human cancer, including 20% to 40% of breast cancer [1-7]. Carcinogen-specific p53 mutation spectra have been described [8]. Germ-line p53 mutations have been reported to be associated with inherited cancer susceptibility in patients with the Li-Fraumeni syndrome which includes breast cancer, soft tissue sarcoma, osteosarcoma, brain tumours, laryngeal cancer, leukaemia, and adrenocortical cancer [9].

Several germ-line polymorphisms representing variable sites in the constitutional genomic DNA have been described for the p53 gene sequence such as a VNTR (variable number tandem repeat) region in intron 1 [10], a 16 bp tandem repeat in intron 3 [11], a *Bst* UI RFLP at codon 72 in exon 4 [12,13], a *Msp* I RFLP in intron 6 [14,15], a *Taq* I RFLP at codon 213 in exon 6 [16], and an Alu sequence at the 3' end of the gene [17]. Three two-allele p53 polymorphisms have been analysed for association with cancer risk. Intron 3 of the p53 gene contains a 16

Address for correspondence: I.B. Runnebaum, Universitäts-Frauenklinik, 89070 Ulm, Germany. Tel.: +49 -731-502 7680, Fax: +49-731-502 7679,
e-mail: ingo.runnebaum@medizin.uni-ulm.de

bp sequence which can occur tandemly duplicated (allele A2 contains the duplication) [11]. In a previous study, we found that the allele frequency of the 16 bp A2 was significantly higher among German ovarian cancer cases [18]. In a Swedish study a significantly lower frequency of the 16 bp A2 allele was observed among colorectal cancer cases compared with controls [19]. The *Bst* UI RFLP recognises a polymorphism at codon 72 which either encodes a proline (CCC, A1) or an arginine (CGC, A2). The *Bst* UI A1A1 genotype was found to be associated with patients who had developed cigarette smoking-induced lung cancer in Japan [20]. Studies in a Swedish population showed similar results for patients with breast cancer but not for patients with lung cancer [21] or colorectal cancer [19]. *Msp* I recognises a polymorphism in intron 6 consisting of either 6 or 8 variable bases [15]. No significant association has been reported for this polymorphism in any cancer population so far. The 16 bp duplication, *Bst* UI, and *Msp* I polymorphisms, as well as pairwise haplotypes involving these three sites were studied in Swedish patients with lung, colorectal, and breast cancer [19,21,22]. Haplotype frequencies of the allele comprising *Bst* UI A1 and 16 bp A1 were found to be associated with lung cancer and colorectal cancer. Haplotypes containing the *Bst* UI A1 allele were more frequently observed in breast cancer patients.

Our group has carried out a hospital-based case-control study of the three p53 polymorphisms in intron 3 (16 bp duplication), in exon 4 (*Bst* UI) and intron 6 (*Msp* I). In this chapter, a novel association of germ-line polymorphic p53 alleles with breast cancer in German women is described.

Viral p53 transduction strategy for gene therapy of breast cancer

Over the past decade, the development of methods for new biological treatments of cancer based on natural host defense mechanisms or the administration of natural mammalian substances has made extraordinary progress through an increased understanding of the cellular immune system as well as through advances of molecular biotechnology. The development of methods for delivering genes into mammalian cells has stimulated great interest in the possibility of treating human disease, including cancer, by gene-based therapy, a concept which has been postulated even before the era of recombinant DNA technology [23,24]. Direct *in situ* introduction of tumour suppressor genes into proliferating tumours could provide an effective therapeutic approach. Retroviral-mediated gene transfer, the current method of choice for clinical gene transfer, offers the potential for stable long-term expression of transduced genes in host cells subsequent to integration of vector DNA into the host genome [1,25].

Transfer of the wild-type p53 tumour suppressor gene is sufficient to suppress some features of the neoplastic phenotype, mostly tumorigenicity of cultured cells derived from various human tumours including colorectal carcinoma, glioblastoma, peripheral neuroepithelioma, prostate cancer, acute lymphoblastic leukaemia, and breast cancer [26-33]. These studies demonstrate that p53 can play a central or even overriding role in the control of cell replication and proliferation. Emerging evidence suggests that the DNA-binding wild-type p53 protein may exert its growth control by regulation of genes related to cell cycle and DNA replication [34,35]. All p53 mutants analysed so far no longer bind to p53-specific DNA binding sites, suggesting that p53 function is dependent at least in part on its role in transcriptional regulation [36-39]. p53, which is expressed in non-cancerous cells at rather low levels, apparently has no vital role in embryonic development and in normal mature cells since p53-deficient mice develop normally [40]. In stressed cells, however, p53 appears to play an important growth-modulating role. Following radiation-induced DNA damage an increase in p53 expression is associated with inhibition of DNA synthesis or apoptosis [41-44]. The cyclin-dependent kinase inhibitor p21$^{WAF1/}$ ^{CIP1} has been shown to be inducible by wild-type p53 [45,46]. Retrovirally mediated introduction of a wild-type copy of the p53 gene into human breast cancer cells has been shown to effectively suppress tumorigenicity in nude mice [32, 33]. p53-based tumour suppression, however, does not necessarily depend on p21$^{WAF1/CIP1}$ induction [47].

In the second part of this chapter, a protocol of repetitive transduction with a wild-type p53 retroviral vector making subsequent selection of a marker gene unnecessary, is presented. This protocol is sufficient to suppress the tumorigenicity of human breast cancer cells containing a p53 point missense mutation.

Materials and methods

Blood and tumour samples

Blood samples were collected from 107 unselected German breast cancer patients at the time of first diagnosis at the Department of Obstetrics and Gynaecology, University of Ulm, during 1993 to 1994. Blood samples of 305 healthy German female blood donors were collected for control at the blood bank of the University of Ulm in 1993. The average age of patients and controls was 55.1 years and 36.9 years, respectively. Genomic DNA was extracted from blood by the phenol chloroform method [48]. Tumour samples were examined by pathologists at the Department of Obstetrics and Gynaecology, University of Ulm. Histopathological malignancy grading was assessed according to accepted standards [49].

PCR amplification and restriction enzyme digest

The analysis of the p53 polymorphic sites was based on the amplification of three fragments encompassing the 16 bp duplication polymorphism in intron 3, the *Bst* UI RFLP in exon 4 at codon 72, and the *Msp* I RFLP in intron 6, using a standard PCR protocol [2]. All PCRs were carried out with 30 cycles each consisting of 1 min of denaturing at 94°C, 1 min of annealing (60°C for 16 bp, 54°C for *Bst* UI and *Msp* I) and 1 min of extension at 72°C. The amplification of the 16 bp

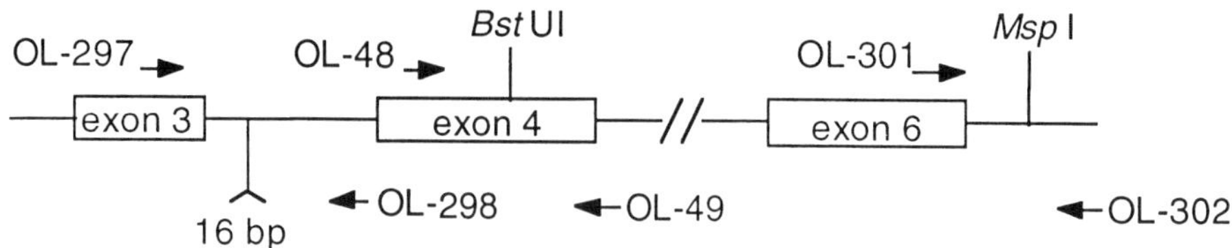

Fig. 1. Scheme of three p53 polymorphic sites and of the oligonucleotide primer location.

duplication polymorphism using the sense primer OL-297 and antisense primer OL-298 resulted in a 119 bp or 135 bp fragment (Fig. 1). PCR products were separated on a high resolution 3% NuSieve agarose gel. The 16 bp A1 allele was defined as the absence of the duplication, according to previous publications [11,18]. The *Bst* UI RFLP sense primer OL-48 and the antisense primer OL-49 amplified a 318 bp PCR product which was digested with *Bst* UI to two fragments of 136 bp and 182 bp (Fig. 1). The *Msp* I RFLP sense primer OL-301 and the antisense primer OL-302 resulted in a 154 bp fragment which after *Msp* I digest produced a 100 bp and a 52 bp fragment (Fig. 1). PCR products were digested to completion with *Bst* UI at 60°C for 2 h or with *Msp* I at 37°C for 2 h. Digests were separated on a 2% agarose gel. The *Bst* UI A1 and the *Msp* I A1 allele were both alleles not presenting the restriction enzyme recognition sites [12,14]. All ethidium bromide-stained fragments were analysed on a UV source using an image analysis system.

Haplotype estimation and statistical analysis

Pairwise and extended haplotype frequencies were estimated based on principles outlined elsewhere [50-52]. The haplotype frequencies were also estimated by using maximum likelihood methods as implemented in the computer software EH (J.D. Terwilliger and J. Ott, 1994). The χ^2 test was used to identify deviations from Hardy-Weinberg proportion [52]. Fisher's exact tests were used to compare the distribution of alleles, haplotypes, and genotype combinations among breast cancer cases and controls. Odds ratios were determined as an estimate of the relative risk. Logistic regression models for the case-control analysis were used to adjust for age. Differences were given as Δ-values. All computations were undertaken using SAS, release 6.11 (SAS Institute, Carey, NC).

Cell lines

Breast cancer cell line MDAMB231 expressing mutant p53 [2] as well as the helper cell lines psi2 and PA317 were obtained from American Type Culture Collection (ATCC). Cells were grown under conditions recommended by ATCC.

Preparation of vectors

The derivation and organisation of the p53 retroviral vector Lhp53RNL used in this study have been described elsewhere [31]. It expresses a wild-type p53 cDNA obtained from Dr. M. Oren. The vector Lhp53RNL expresses the human p53 cDNA from the Moloney murine leukaemia virus 5' LTR and the bacterial neomycin phosphotransferase gene from the Rous sarcoma virus LTR. The similar retrovirus construct pLLRNL containing the firefly luciferase gene instead of the p53 cDNA was used for negative control. Control vector LZRNL has been described elsewhere [53]. Techniques used for production and titration of retroviral vectors were similar to those reported elsewhere [31]. Clones producing high titers were identified by titration of producer cell supernatant on 208F cells and the production of p53 was determined by immunoprecipitation [33].

Transduction, analysis of ß-galactosidase activity

For bulk transduction of breast carcinoma cells, supernatant media from cloned producer cells containing $2x10^4$ to $5x10^4$ colony-forming units/ml of the retrovirus and 8 µg/ml of Polybrene (Sigma) were used. The supernatant media (20 ml on 10-cm tissue culture plates) were changed every 4 hours until a multiplicity of infection (moi) of 2 was reached. Cells were then kept in regular non-selective medium for at least 24 to 48 hours. The susceptibility of MDAMB231 cells to transduction was determined using LZRNL at a moi of 2 followed by cytochemical detection of ß-galactosidase activity 48 hours after transduction [53]. MDAMB231 cells to be G418-selected were transduced by a standard protocol with a moi of 0.005 followed by a medium change after 48 hours to a G418-containing medium (800 µg/ml). G418-selected cells were expanded under selection for 4 to 6 weeks.

Growth rate and anchorage-independent growth

Lhp53RNL-, LLRNL- and mock-transduced MDAMB231 cells (moi 2) were plated in triplicate at densities of $5x10^2$, 10^3, $5x10^3$, 10^4, $5x10^4$ and 10^5 cells on 24-well, 6-well or 10-cm plates. Cells removed from monolayers by EDTA were counted periodically in a Coulter counter until they reached confluence. Anchorage-independent growth was examined by established methods, plating in triplicate viability-tested cell suspensions in 0.35% agar in DME supplemented with 10% fetal calf serum on top of a 0.55% agar basal layer. Colony formation was assessed after 2 weeks when $5x10^3$ and $5x10^4$ cells were plated or after 4 weeks when $2x10^2$, $2x10^3$ cells were plated and supplemented again after 2 weeks with 0.35% agar in DME with 10% fetal calf serum.

Tumorigenicity

Transduced or control MDAMB231 cells were harvested from culture without trypsin treatment, resuspended and injected subcutaneously in volumes of 100 µl containing 5×10^6 or 10^7 cells into the shoulders and flanks of female nu/nu mice 4 to 5 weeks of age. Transduced and untransduced cells were injected into different sites of the same mouse or separately into different mice. Viability of cells was established by trypan blue exclusion prior to injection and approximate tumour volumes were determined from measurements of tumour size *in vivo*.

Results

p53 genotype and haplotype analysis

Genotype analysis was performed for three polymorphic sites in the p53 gene of 107 German women with breast cancer and 305 healthy control women. The genotype distribution in patients and controls did not deviate from expected Hardy-Weinberg frequencies at any of the three sites tested. The *Msp* I A1 allele was found to be associated with an increased approximate relative risk for breast cancer in German women with an age-adjusted odds ratio (OR) of 1.57 and a 95% confidence interval (95% CI) of 0.84-2.94. The *Msp* I A1 allele was observed more frequently in the breast cancer patients than in controls, although the difference was statistically not significant (p=0.075). The 16 bp A2 allele was more frequent in breast cancer patients with an age-adjusted OR of 1.31 and a 95% CI of 0.71-2.42. The allele frequency of 16 bp A2 was 0.16 in breast cancer patients and 0.12 in controls. The difference, however, was not statistically significant (p=0.161). The genotype distribution of the *Bst* UI polymorphism did not differ in cases and controls (p=0.977). In the majority of the individuals genotyped, the rare 16 bp A2 allele was in apparent linkage disequilibrium with the rare *Msp* I A1 allele, and the frequent 16 bp A1 was in apparent linkage disequilibrium with the frequent *Msp* I A2. This phenomenon was observed in 105/107 (98%) of breast cancer cases and in 297/305 (97%) of controls. Surprisingly, this association was independent of the *Bst* UI site in exon 4, which lies between the other two loci (Fig. 1).

At all three polymorphic sites, the breast cancer patients were more frequently heterozygous than the control individuals: *Msp* I A1A2 (∆=9%, p=0.046; ∆=difference), 16 bp A1A2 (∆=6%, p=0.23) and *Bst* UI A1A2 (∆=5%, p=0.40). Decreased frequencies of the homozygous genotypes *Msp* I A2A2 (∆=9%), 16 bp A1A1 (∆=7%), and *Bst* UI A2A2 (∆=3%) were observed in the breast cancer cases while the frequencies of the homozygous genotypes *Msp* I A1A1, *Bst* UI A1A1 and 16 bp A2A2 were similar between cases and controls.

For each individual, genotype results of all three polymorphisms were analysed together as a combination. A significant difference (Fisher's exact test, p=0.017) was found between patients and controls for such genotype combinations. The triple heterozygotes of the three polymorphisms were more frequent in the breast cancer patients (25%) than in the control group (17%), with an age-adjusted OR of 2.01 and a 95% CI of 1.02-3.94. The distribution of the other two common genotype combinations (16 bp A1A1-*Bst* UI A2A2-*Msp* I A2A2 and 16 bp A1A1-*Bst* UI A2A1-*Msp* I A2A2) were also different in the two groups. Both combinations were found at a lower frequency in the breast cancer group than in controls. The haplotype frequency differences were 4% for the 16 bp A1A1-*Bst* UI A2A2-*Msp* I A2A2 combination and 3% for the 16 bp A1A1-*Bst* UI A2A1-*Msp* I A2A2 combination (Fisher's exact test, p=0.161).

Allele frequencies of the three p53 polymorphisms were correlated with the histological malignancy grade. Patients with low grade tumours (G1, G2) tended to show a higher frequency of the rare alleles *Msp* I A1, 16 bp A2 and *Bst* UI A1 than patients with G3 tumours, who did not show differences in the allele frequencies of the three polymorphic sites compared to the healthy control group. The *Bst* UI A1 allele was slightly more frequent in the subgroups with tumours of higher differentiation (G1 group: Fisher's exact test, p=0.034). Alleles in the histological subgroups were in Hardy-Weinberg proportion.

Pairwise haplotype frequencies were estimated for all possible combinations of the three polymorphisms in cases and controls. A significantly different distribution of the *Bst* UI-*Msp* I haplotype was found between breast cancer patients and healthy individuals (Fisher's exact test, p=0.041). Haplotypes carrying the *Msp* I A1 were estimated to be more frequently present in the breast cancer group (14.3% *Bst* UI A1-*Msp* I A1 and 1.1% *Bst* UI A2-*Msp* I A1) than in the control group (10.8% *Bst* UI A1-*Msp* I A1 and 0% *Bst* UI A2-*Msp* I A1). Accordingly, the frequencies of the haplotypes with the *Msp* I A2 were lower in the breast cancer group. In the combination of *Bst* UI-16 bp, the differences in haplotype frequencies (breast cancer group: 13.7% *Bst* UI A1-16 bp A2 and 2.2% *Bst* UI A2-16 bp A2; control group: 11.5% in 1-2 allele and 0.6% in 2-2 allele) were not statistically significant (Fisher's exact test, p=0.160). In the combination of *Msp* I-16 bp, the differences in the haplotype frequencies of *Msp* I A1-16 bp A2 were not statistically significant (Δ=4.2%, p=0.131, Fisher's exact test).

The estimation of the haplotype frequencies was extended to all three polymorphic sites for cases and controls. The estimated haplotype frequencies in the two groups differed significantly (Fisher's exact test, p=0.029). In the 16 bp-*Bst* UI-*Msp* I haplotypes, the frequency of 16 bp A2-*Bst* UI A1-*Msp* I A1 (2-1-1) and 2-2-1 was higher in the breast cancer group (13.7% for 2-1-1 and 1.1% for 2-2-1) than in the healthy control group (10.8% for 2-1-1 and 0% for 2-2-1). The extended haplotype estimation revealed that haplotypes comprising 16 bp A2-*Msp* I A1 were the more frequent haplotypes in the breast cancer patients.

Retrovirally mediated p53 gene transduction

The susceptibility of MDAMB231 breast cancer cells to transduction with the retroviral vector system used in this study was determined with the recombinant virus LZRNL transducing the lacZ reporter gene. Multiple subsequent exposures of MDAMB231 with amphotropic LZRNL freshly harvested from

PA317 producer cell line cultures of which virus production was titered in parallel were carried out until a multiplicity of infection of 2 was reached. In approximately 90% of the exposed cell population this procedure resulted in cytochemically detectable ß-galactosidase activity when tested 48 hours as well as 1 week after transduction using non-selective media.

Reduction of the cellular growth rate

To determine effects of wild-type p53 expression on the cellular growth rate, identical numbers of exponentially growing MDAMB231 cells were transduced at a multiplicity of infection (moi) of 2 with either Lhp53RNL or control virus, or the cells were mock-infected. Trypan blue cell exclusion revealed no significant differences in the viability of the cells immediately after transduction with the two vectors compared with mock-transduced cells. Lhp53RNL-transduced cells showed a significantly reduced growth rate compared with that of the mock-transduced or LLRNL-transduced cells (Fig. 2). Lhp53RNL-transduced MDAMB231 cells had a doubling time of 40.2 hours compared to 30.0 and 31.9 hours of mock-transduced or LLRNL-transduced MDAMB231 cells, respectively.

Suppression of anchorage-independent growth

The tumorigenic properties of MDAMB231 were also examined by determining the ability of cells to grow under anchorage-independent conditions. Cells were transduced with either LLRNL or Lhp53RNL at a moi of 2, applying the described protocol. By trypan blue exclusion more than 90% of the transduced cells remained viable after transduction. Colonies consisting of more than 100 cells were counted. Since colonies formed by Lhp53RNL-transduced cells did not expand over more than 30 cells per colony, smaller colonies were considered positive. The ability of Lhp53RNL-transduced MDAMB231 cells to form colonies in semi-solid medium was reduced 20-fold compared with LLRNL or mock-transduced cells (Table 1).

Table 1. Efficiency of anchorage-independent colony formation of Lhp53RNL-transduced MDAMB231 breast cancer cells

No. of cells seeded/weeks	No. of colonies Lhp53RNL	No. of colonies LLRNL	No. of colonies uninfected
50 000 / 2	60	1210	1193
5 000 / 2	2	91	86
2 000 / 4	1	49	53
200 / 4	0	9	12

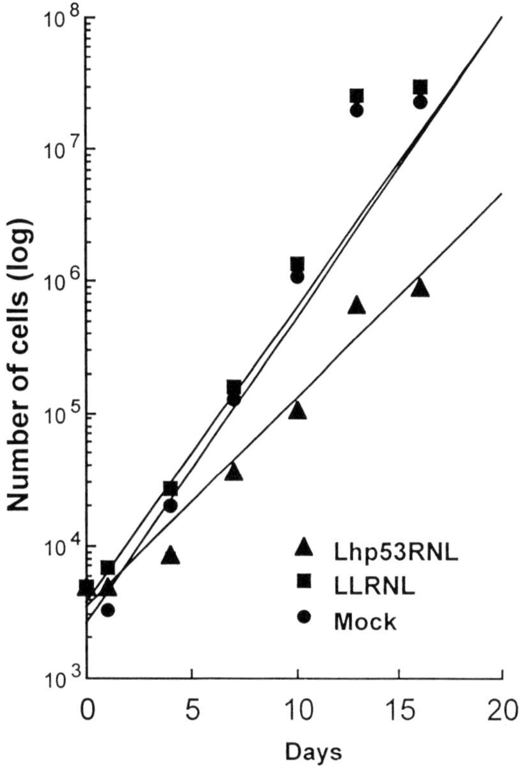

Fig. 2. Effect of wt p53 on the growth rate of MDAMB231 after infection with Lhp53RNL. Two days after infection, 5×10^3 cells were replated in triplicate (day 0). Cell numbers were determined in a Coulter counter after trypsinization beginning on day 1 and repeated every 3 days until the control cultures (infected with LLRNL or uninfected) reached confluence. Mean cell numbers from one representative experiment are indicated.

Suppression of tumorigenicity

The effect of transfer of the wild-type p53 gene by simple retroviral bulk transduction on the tumorigenic properties of breast cancer cells containing only a mutant p53 gene was tested by subcutaneous injection of G418-non-selected cells into immunodeficient nude mice. As described elsewhere [54], the parental MDAMB231 cells were highly tumorigenic. Palpable tumours appeared as early as 1 week after injection in nude mice injected with 5×10^6 and 10^7 parental MDAMB231 cells. To examine the effect of wild-type p53 expression on tumour formation, 5×10^6 and 10^7 mock-transduced, LLRNL or Lhp53RNL-transduced cells were injected subcutaneously. The time of appearance and the volumes of the resulting tumours were determined (Fig. 3). Tumours induced by 10^7 mock-transduced cells became readily palpable one week after injection while

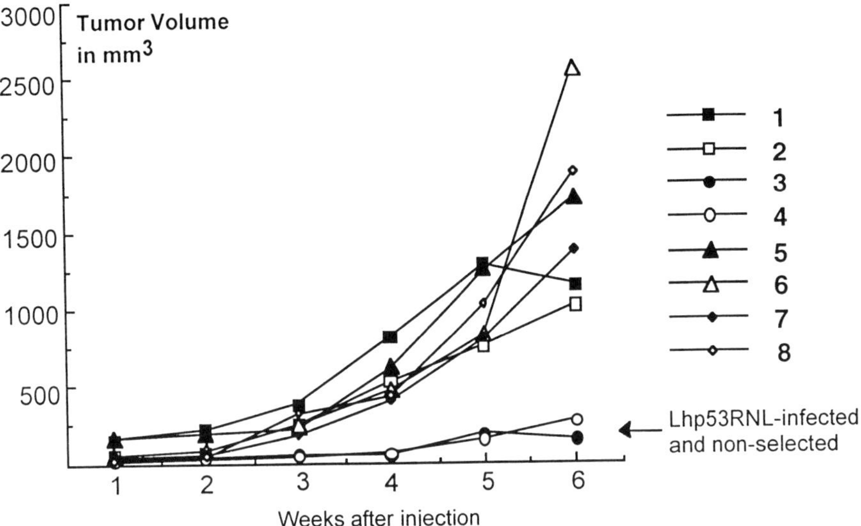

Fig. 3. Effect of Lhp53RNL bulk infection without selection on tumorigenicity of MDAMB231. Volumes of subcutaneous tumours in nude mice were followed for 6 weeks after implantation of 5×10^6 and 10^7 cells which were mock-infected or bulk-infected with either LLRNL or Lhp53RNL or infected with Lhp53RNL and subsequently neo-selected. Tumour sizes were measured every week. Mean volumes from three tumour sites are plotted: (1) 10^7 MDAMB231, (2) 5×10^6 MDAMB231, (3) 10^7 MDAMB231, Lhp53RNL bulk-infected, (4) 5×10^6 MDAMB231, Lhp53RNL bulk-infected, (5) 10^7 MDAMB231, LLRNL bulk-infected, (6) 5×10^6 MDAMB231, LLRNL bulk-infected, (7) 10^7 MDAMB231, Lhp53RNL infected and G418-selected, (8) 5×10^6 MDAMB231, Lhp53RNL infected and G418-selected.

smaller masses were found at the same time in sites injected with 5×10^6 cells. By 6 weeks after injection, large tumours of similar size formed at sites receiving both doses of cells. Similar results were obtained in recipient nude mice injected with cells bulk-transduced with LLRNL virus at a moi of 2. In contrast, we were unable to detect growing tumours in nude mice injected with either dose, 10^7 or 5×10^6 cells, transduced with Lhp53RNL virus at a moi of 2. In a few animals only small nodules had formed. Histological examination of this tissue detected granulomatous tissue and no proliferating tumour cells, as shown previously [33]. For long-term follow-up mice were injected with Lhp53RNL-transduced and non-selected cells only. No tumour formation became apparent during 12 weeks following injection, indicating efficient suppression of the tumorigenic potential of the Lhp53RNL-exposed and non-selected breast cancer cell population.

MDAMB231 cells were also transduced by a standard protocol with a moi of 0.005 followed by stringent G418 selection. Ten to 12 days of exposure to 800 µg/ml of geneticin led to elimination of untransduced cells. Remaining clones of transduced cells were expanded in the presence of the G418 for 4 to 6 weeks to reach cell numbers required for tumorigenicity testing. With regard to the cell number, the resulting clones were pooled instead of separately expanding single clones. Recipient nude mice developed tumours from Lhp53RNL-transduced and G418-selected cells in a similar time frame as when injected with cells from the parent MDAMB231 cell line.

Discussion

Genotype analysis of breast cancer patients and healthy control subjects revealed differences in the allelic distribution of the 16 bp polymorphism in intron 3 and the *Msp* I polymorphism in intron 6 of the p53 gene. The distribution of the three polymorphisms was in Hardy-Weinberg proportion. Two alleles, *Msp* I A1 and 16 bp A2, were found to be associated with an increased odds ratio associated with breast cancer. By contrast, the allelic distribution of the *Bst* UI polymorphism did not differ between cases and controls. These observations were supported by a pairwise haplotype estimation. Therefore, our results suggest that the *Msp* I A1 or 16 bp A2 alleles may be associated with elevated breast cancer risk.

The genotypic combinations of all three polymorphic sites were analysed in cases and controls to search for combinations overrepresented in breast cancer cases. In the breast cancer patients, the heterozygotes for 16 bp A1A2 and *Msp* I A1A2 were more frequent (28% vs. 20%) as compared to controls. The triple heterozygote combinations revealed 16 bp A2-*Bst* UI A1-*Msp* I A1 (2-1-1) and 16 bp A2-*Bst* UI A2-*Msp* I A1 (2-2-1) as haplotypes overrepresented in the breast cancer cases. This estimation suggested that the *Msp* I A1 and 16 bp A2 constitute haplotypes that may be potential risk factors for breast cancer in German women.

The rare 16 bp A2 allele in intron 3 was found in combination with the rare intron 6 *Msp* I A1 allele. In addition, the frequent 16 bp A1 was found together with the frequent *Msp* I A2. This phenomenon was observed in 98% of the breast cancer patients and controls, indicating a linkage disequilibrium for these polymorphic intragenic markers. The association of 16 bp A2 and *Msp* I A2 was independent of the type of the *Bst* UI site located in exon 4. One interpretation consistent with this result is that the *Bst* UI polymorphism may be a late genetic event associated with either a 16 bp A2 - *Msp* I A2 or a 16 bp A1 - *Msp* I A1 haplotype.

All three polymorphisms tested in this study have also been tested in a Swedish population with and without breast cancer [22]. The allele frequencies of the polymorphisms in our control population were very similar to those of the Swedish control population, allowing a comparison of the two breast cancer patient samples. An adjustment of the odds ratios for age was not presented in the Swedish study since the majority of the controls consisted of newborns, a control group with limited value by epidemiological standards. The data of the Swedish and our German study cannot be directly compared since the average age of the Swedish cancer group has not been given. An apparent difference between the Swedish and the German cancer group was the distribution of histological differentiation. In the Swedish breast cancer group as opposed to our own patient series a large number of patients had well differentiated tumours. *Bst* UI A1 was more frequently present in Swedish patients while 16 bp A2 and *Msp* I A1 were more frequently found in the German sample. Our data do not support the hypothesis of a functional insufficiency of the proline encoded by *Bst* UI A1 allele. The prevalence of 16 bp A2 and *Msp* I A1 alleles in the German breast cancer samples argues for a linkage disequilibrium rather than an alliance between the intronic variations and the p53 gene function.

In the pairwise haplotype estimation of German and Swedish breast cancer patients different allele combinations were calculated to be more frequent than in control subjects. The more frequent haplotypes in Swedish breast cancer patients contained the *Bst* UI AI allele in all combinations [22]. In the German breast cancer patients either the 16 bp A2 or the *Msp* I A1 alleles in any of the haplotype combinations were calculated to be more frequent than in control subjects. Extension of the haplotype calculation to all three variable sites confirmed the haplotypes comprising 16 bp A2 and *Msp* I A1 as the risk haplotypes in the German breast cancer patients. The extended haplotype associated with Swedish colorectal cancer patients was deduced from genotype data to be 16 bp A1-*Bst* UI A1-*Msp* I A1 [19]. Extended haplotype data cannot be related to data from other populations since extended haplotype estimations have not been performed in published studies on p53 polymorphisms so far.

Patients with histologically well differentiated tumours have been reported to carry the rare *Bst* UI A1 allele more frequently than patients with undifferentiated breast or lung cancer [20,22]. A similar trend was observed for *Bst* UI A1 in our patient group with well differentiated tumours. In addition, the potential risk alleles 16 bp A2 and *Msp* I A1 identified in this study were also more frequent in patients with low-grade tumours.

p53 gene transduction

We have established an efficient and simple protocol for retrovirus-mediated tumour suppressor gene delivery into cancer cells. This study has demonstrated potent suppression of tumorigenicity of MDAMB231 breast cancer cells by transfer of the wild-type p53 tumour suppressor gene. MDAMB231 was chosen for displaying a number of features characteristic of primary human breast cancer. In about 30% of breast cancers, p53 protein accumulation has been observed and has been correlated with p53 gene mutations, histological dedifferentiation, lack of oestrogen and/or progesterone receptors, high aggressiveness and shortened patient survival [55-57]. MDAMB231 expresses a mutant p53 showing accumulation of the gene product with an extended half-life of 7 h [2,33]. This cell line is derived from a highly undifferentiated adenocarcinoma of the breast, expresses no detectable oestrogen or progesterone receptors and is capable of forming tumours in nude mice [54,58]. In addition to a point missense mutation in the p53 gene, MDAMB231 contains an activated K-ras oncogene and expresses high levels of the growth factor IGF-I, consistent with the concept of a multistep development of the breast cancer phenotype [32,59,60].

The development of the neoplastic phenotype in most sporadic human cancers is thought to result from cooperation between a number of activated oncogenes and the loss of activity of tumour suppressor genes. Correcting just one such defect by transfer of wild-type p53 alleles into different cell lines has been demonstrated in this and other studies to be sufficient to suppress at least some features of the tumour phenotype. Such cell lines were derived from a variety of human tumours including colorectal carcinoma, glioblastoma, peripheral neuroepithelioma, prostate cancer, breast cancer, and acute lymphoblastic leukaemia [26-32]. Suppression of tumorigenicity in immunosuppressed mice was most consistently observed in these systems. Lhp53RNL transduction *trans*-dominantly suppressed tumorigenicity in MDAMB231 harbouring multiple genetic alterations beyond a p53 gene mutation. Since transduction was carried out at a moi of 2, most transduced MDAMB231 cells can be expected to contain a single copy of the wild-type p53 provirus. Under these conditions, efficient suppression of the tumorigenicity of MDAMB231 suggested that the transduced wild-type p53 was providing tumour suppressor function to a cell expressing an endogenous loss-of-function p53 mutant. Alternatively, the retrovirally transduced wild-type p53 allele could be exerting a dominant effect over a gain-of-function growth stimulatory activity of the endogenous mutant gene. In another recent study, equal transcription of wild-type and mutant p53 from bicistronic vectors resulted in the dominance of the wild-type form with regard to cell growth [61]. Similarly, transformation of REFs by gain-of-function mutant Val^{135} plus activated ras was inhibited by coexpression of wild-type p53 [62]. These observations demonstrated that wild-type p53 can exercise a *trans*-dominant effect over transforming p53 mutants.

Selection of p53-transduced or transfected breast cancer cells with a selectable marker together with p53 in other studies has resulted in a majority of clones not expressing the p53 transgene [30,32]. Similarly, injection of nude mice with MDAMB231, Lhp53RNL-transduced at a low moi and selected *in vitro* with G418 for 4 to 6 weeks, resulted in the formation of tumours at the same time and of the same size as seen after injection of either mock-transduced parental or LLRNL-transduced cells. It is possible that the tumours were derived from cells in which expression of the p53 cDNA had been lost by genetic or even epigenetic mechanisms and which were selected with great efficiency during growth in G418-selective medium. However, when MDAMB231 cells were not selected after bulk transduction with Lhp53RNL at a moi of 2, efficient suppression of the tumorigenic phenotype occurred, indicating that the majority of cells had received a functional copy of wild-type p53. Long-term follow-up after injection into nude mice for 12 weeks suggested that the wild-type p53 gene was stably expressed. Stable expression of a reporter gene product (interleukin-2 receptor, IL2R) unrelated to growth properties of the cell has been observed in CFT-1 cells (cystic fibrosis epithelial cell line) for at least one year following multiple infections with an amphotropic retrovirus in the absence of G418 selection [63]. The IL2R retrovirus also contained a neomycin phosphotransferase gene as a dominant selectable marker. A decline in IL2R reporter gene expression was observed under constant selection pressure for expression of the neo^R gene as in our study where neo-selected cells formed tumours. Stable expression even of a growth inhibiting gene may be better maintained without selection. Retrovirus-mediated gene transfer offering stable expression of transduced genes based on integration of vector DNA into the host genome may well be the vector of choice in clinical applications in the future, especially with the recent development of high titer pseudotype retrovirus preparations, e.g. using the G protein of vesicular stomatitis virus as an envelope [64].

Conclusions

This chapter demonstrates how basic science knowledge of the p53 gene may become applicable to patient care:

1) p53 haplotype analysis may be helpful in individual breast cancer risk assessment. We have identified two alleles (16 bp A2 and *Msp* I A1) that appear to be overrepresented in patients with breast cancer. Certain p53 alleles appear to modify the individual breast cancer risk. In combination with classic epidemiological data, this approach could lead to the definition of p53 alleles predisposing to increased breast cancer susceptibility. Assessing the p53 polymorphism status may eventually assist in counseling women regarding their individual breast cancer risk.

2) Virally mediated p53 gene transfer may develop into novel adjuvant therapeutic intervention strategies in combination with established therapy methods. This chapter summarises encouraging experimental data for the development of gene therapy. The ability of a genetic correction of only one of multiple genetic defects in tumour cells to suppress aspects of the tumour phenotype is surprising, and the mechanisms are still not well understood. The presented protocol was developed as an approach to efficiently reconstitute wild-type p53 growth control in tumour cells *in vivo*. Our present observations, together with the results of previous work, suggest that restoration of wild-type p53 gene expression, even in cells already containing activated oncogenes or defective tumour suppressor genes, holds great promise in the development of a p53 gene-directed treatment for some forms of human tumours including breast cancer.

Acknowledgements

The author wishes to thank the colleagues who made possible the projects of which the data are summarised in this chapter and published separately elsewhere: in the polymorphism project, Shan Wang (Molecular Biology Laboratory, Department of Obstetrics and Gynaecology, University of Ulm); for helpful discussions Rolf Kreienberg (Director of the Department of Obstetrics and Gynaecology, University of Ulm), Timothy Rebbeck (Department of Biostatistics and Epidemiology, University of Pennsylvania, School of Medicine, Philadelphia, PA, USA) and Dirk G. Kieback (Department of Obstetrics and Gynaecology, Baylor College of Medicine, Houston, TX, USA); for providing buffy coats Werner Körner (Blood Bank, University of Ulm); for providing histopathological data Wolfgang Böhm (Department of Obstetrics and Gynaecology, University of Ulm); for the support in gene transfer technology Jing-Kuan Yee (previously University of California, San Diego, CA, USA), Theodore Friedmann (Director of the Gene Therapy Program, University of California, San Diego, CA, USA) and Saraswati Sukumar (previously The Salk Institute, San Diego, CA, USA, now Director of the Basic Breast Cancer Research Program, Johns Hopkins University, Baltimore, MD, USA). The support of the Deutsche Forschungsgemeinschaft (DFG RU476/1-1, RU476/ 1-2 and RU476/2-1) and the institutional funds (P.234 and P.317) from the Klinikumsvorstand of the University of Ulm granted to the author are also acknowledged.

References

1   Hollstein M, Sidransky D, Vogelstein B, Harris CC. p53 mutations in human cancers. Science 1991; 253: 49-53
2   Runnebaum IB, Nagarajan M, Bowman M, Soto D, Sukumar S. Mutations in p53 as potential molecular markers for human breast cancer. Proc Natl Acad Sci USA 1991; 88: 10657-61
3   Varley JM, Brammar WJ, Lane DP, Swallow JE, Dolan C, Walker RA. Loss of chromosome 17p13 sequences and mutation of p53 in human breast carcinomas. Oncogene 1991; 6: 413-21
4   Coles C, Condie A, Chetty U, Steel CM, Evans HJ, Prosser J. p53 mutations in breast cancer. Cancer Res 1992; 52: 5291-8
5   Osborne RJ, Merlo GR, Mitsudomi T et al. Mutations in the p53 gene in primary human breast cancers. Cancer Res 1991; 51: 6194-8
6   Sommer SS, Cunningham J, McGovern RM et al. Pattern of p53 gene mutations in breast cancers of women of the Midwestern United States. J Natl Cancer Inst 1992; 84: 246-52
7   Bergh J, Norberg T, Sjögren S, Lindgren A, Holmberg L. Complete sequencing of the p53 gene provides prognostic information in breast cancer patients, particularly in relation to adjuvant systemic therapy and radiotherapy. Nature Med 1995; 1: 1029-34
8   Harris CC. p53: At the crossroads of molecular carcinogenesis and risk assessment. Science 1993; 262: 1980-1
9   Malkin D, Li FP, Strong LC, Fraumeni JJ et al. Germ line p53 mutations in a familial syndrome of breast cancer, sarcomas, and other neoplasms. Science 1990; 250: 1233-8

10 Hahn M, Serth J, Fislage R et al. Polymerase chain reaction detection of a highly polymorphic VNTR segment in intron 1 of the human p53 gene. Clin Chem 1993; 39: 549-50

11 Lazar V, Hazard F, Bertin F, Janin N, Bellet D, Bressac B. Simple sequence repeat polymorphism within the p53 gene. Oncogene 1993; 8: 1703-5

12 Harris N, Brill E, Shohat O et al. Molecular basis for heterogeneity of the human p53 protein. Mol Cell Biol 1986; 6: 4650-6

13 Matlashewski GJ, Tuck S, Pim D, Lamb P, Schneider J, Crawford LV. Primary structure polymorphism at amino acid residue 72 of human p53. Mol Cell Biol 1987; 7: 961-3

14 McDaniel T, Carbone D, Takahashi T et al. The MspI polymorphism in intron 6 of p53 (TP53) detected by digestion of PCR products. Nucleic Acids Res 1991; 19: 4796

15 Peller S, Kopilova Y, Slutzki S, Halevy A, Kvitko K, Rotter V. A novel polymorphism in intron 6 of the human p53 gene: a possible association with cancer predisposition and susceptibility. DNA Cell Biol 1995; 14: 983-90

16 Carbone D, Chiba I, Mitsudomi T. Polymorphism at codon 213 within the p53 gene. Oncogene 1991; 6: 1691-2

17 Futreal PA, Barrett JC, Wiseman RW. An Alu polymorphism intragenic to the TP53 gene. Nucleic Acids Res 1991; 19: 6977

18 Runnebaum IB, Tong XW, Konig R et al. p53-based blood test for p53PIN3 and risk for sporadic ovarian cancer. Lancet 1995; 345: 994

19 Sjalander A, Birgander R, Athlin L et al. P53 germ line haplotypes associated with increased risk for colorectal cancer. Carcinogenesis 1995; 16: 1461-4

20 Kawajiri K, Nakachi K, Imai K, Watanabe J, Hayashi S. Germ line polymorphisms of p53 and CYP1A1 genes involved in human lung cancer. Carcinogenesis 1993; 14: 1085-9

21 Birgander R, Sjalander A, Rannug A et al. P53 polymorphisms and haplotypes in lung cancer. Carcinogenesis 1995; 16: 2233-6

22 Sjalander A, Birgander R, Hallmans G et al. p53 polymorphisms and haplotypes in breast cancer. Carcinogenesis 1996; 17: 1313-6

23 Friedmann T, Roblin R. Gene therapy for human genetic disease? Science 1972; 175: 949-55

24 Friedmann T. Progress toward human gene therapy. Science 1989; 244: 1275-80

25 de Frommentel CC, Soussi T. TP53 tumor suppressor gene: A model for investigating human mutagenesis. Genes Chrom Cancer 1992; 4: 1-15

26 Baker SJ, Markowitz S, Fearon ER, Willson JK, Vogelstein B. Suppression of human colorectal carcinoma cell growth by wild-type p53. Science 1990; 249: 912-5

27 Mercer WE, Shields MT, Amin M et al. Negative growth regulation in a glioblastoma tumor cell line that conditionally expresses human wild-type p53. Proc Natl Acad Sci USA 1990; 87: 6166-70

28 Chen YM, Chen PL, Arnaiz N, Goodrich D, Lee WH. Expression of wild-type p53 in human A673 cells suppresses tumorigenicity but not growth rate. Oncogene 1991; 6: 1799-805

29 Isaacs WB, Carter BS, Ewing CM. Wild-type p53 suppresses growth of human prostate cancer cells containing mutant p53 alleles. Cancer Res 1991; 51: 4716-20

30 Casey G, Lo HM, Lopez ME, Vogelstein B, Stanbridge EJ. Growth suppression of human breast cancer cells by the introduction of a wild-type p53 gene. Oncogene 1991; 6: 1791-7

31 Cheng J, Yee JK, Yeargin J, Friedmann T, Haas M. Suppression of acute lymphoblastic leukemia by the human wild-type p53 gene. Cancer Res 1992; 52: 222-6

32 Wang NP, To H, Lee W-H, Lee EY-HP. Tumor suppressor activity of RB and p53 genes in human breast carcinoma cells. Oncogene 1993; 8: 279-88

33 Runnebaum IB, Yee J-K, Kieback DG, Sukumar S, Friedmann T. Wild-type p53 suppresses the malignant phenotype in breast cancer cells containing mutant p53 alleles. Anticancer Res 1994; 14: 1137-44

34 Lin D, Shields MT, Ullrich SJ, Appella E, Mercer WE. Growth arrest induced by wild-type p53 protein blocks cells prior to or near the restriction point in late G1 phase. Proc Natl Acad Sci USA 1992; 89: 9210-4

35 Mercer WE, Shields MT, Lin D, Appella E, Ullrich SJ. Growth suppression induced by wild-type p53 protein is accompanied by selective down-regulation of proliferating-cell nuclear antigen expression. Proc Natl Acad Sci USA 1991; 88: 1958-62

36 Funk WD, Pak DT, Karas RH, Wright WE, Shay JW. A transcriptionally active DNA-binding site for human p53 protein complexes. Mol Cell Biol 1992; 12: 2866-71

37 Vogelstein B, Kinzler KW. p53 function and dysfunction. Cell 1992; 70: 523-6

38 El-Deiry WS, Kern SE, Pietenpol JA, Kinzler KW, Vogelstein B. Definition of a consensus binding site for p53. Nature Genetics 1992; 1: 45-9

39 Kern SE, Pietenpol JA, Thiagalingam S, Seymour A, Kinzler KW, Vogelstein B. Oncogenic forms of p53 inhibit p53-regulated gene expression. Science 1992; 256: 827-30

40 Donehower L, Harvey M, Slagle B et al. Mice deficient for p53 are developmentally normal but susceptible to spontaneous tumors. Nature 1992; 356: 215-21

41 Zhan Q, Carrier F, Fornace AJJ. Induction of cellular p53 activity by DNA-damaging agents and growth arrest. Mol Cell Biol 1993; 13: 4242-50

42 Kastan MB, Onyekwere O, Sidransky D, Vogelstein B, Craig RW. Participation of p53 protein in the cellular response to DNA damage. Cancer Res 1991; 51: 6304-11

43 Kastan MB, Zhan Q, el Deiry W et al. A mammalian cell cycle checkpoint pathway utilizing p53 and GADD45 is defective in ataxia-telangiectasia. Cell 1992; 71: 587-97

44 Kuerbitz SJ, Plunkett BS, Walsh WV, Kastan MB. Wild-type p53 is a cell cycle checkpoint determinant following irradiation. Proc Natl Acad Sci USA 1992; 89: 7491-5

45 Harper JW, Adami GR, Wei N, Keyomarsi K, Elledge SJ. The p21 cdk-interacting protein Cip1 is a potent inhibitor of G1 cyclin-dependent kinases. Cell 1993; 75: 805-16

46 El-Deiry WS, Takino T, Velculescu VE et al. WAF1, a potential mediator of p53 tumor suppression. Cell 1993; 75: 817-25

47 Runnebaum IB, Wang S, Kreienberg R. Retrovirally mediated wild-type p53 restores S phase modulation without inducing *WAF1* mRNA in breast carcinoma cells containing mutant p53. J Cell Biochem 1995; 59: 538-44

48 Gustafson S, Proper JA, Bowie EJ, Sommer SS. Parameters affecting the yield of DNA from human blood. Anal Biochem 1987; 165: 294-9

49 Trojani M. A colour atlas of breast histopathology, English edition. London, New York, Tokyo, Melbourne, Madras: Chapman and Hall, 1991

50 Hill WG. Estimation of linkage disequilibrium in randomly mating populations. Heredity 1974; 33: 229-39

51 Bennett JH, Oertel CR. The approach to a random association of genotypes with random mating. J Theor Biol 1965; 9: 67-76

52 Weir BS. Genetic data analysis. Sunderland, MA: Sinauer Associates Inc. Publishers, 1990

53 Xu L, Yee J-K, Wolf JA, Friedmann T. Factors affecting long-term stability of Moloney murine leukemia virus-based vectors. Virology 1989; 171: 331-41

54 Cailleau R, Young R, Olive M, Reeves WJ, Jr. Breast tumor cell lines from pleural effusions. J Natl Canc Inst 1974; 53: 661-74

55 Thor AD, Moore D, Edgerton SM et al. Accumulation of p53 tumor suppressor gene protein: an independent marker of prognosis in breast cancers. J Natl Cancer Inst 1992; 84: 845-55

56 Mazars R, Spinardi L, Ben CM, Simony LJ, Jeanteur P, Theillet C. p53 mutations occur in aggressive breast cancer. Cancer Res 1992; 52: 3918-23

57 Isola J, Visakorpi T, Holli K, Kallioniemi OP. Association of overexpression of tumor suppressor protein p53 with rapid cell proliferation and poor prognosis in node-negative breast cancer patients. J Natl Cancer Inst 1992; 84: 1109-14

58 Engel L, Young N. Human breast carcinoma cells in continuous culture: A review. Cancer Res 1978; 38: 4327-39

59   Kozma SC, Bogaard ME, Buser K et al. The human c-kirsten *ras* gene is activated by a novel mutation in codon 13 in the breast carcinoma cell line MDAMB-231. Nucleic Acids Res 1987; 15: 5963-71

60   Huff KK, Kaufmann D, Gabbay KH, Spencer EM, Lippman ME, Dickson RB. Secretion of an insulin-like growth factor-I-related protein by human breast cancer cells. Cancer Res 1986; 46: 4613-9

61   Frebourg T, Sadelain M, Ng Y-S, Kassel J, Friend SH. Equal transcription of wild-type and mutant p53 using bicistronic vectors results in the wild-type phenotype. Cancer Res 1994; 54: 878-81

62   Finlay CA, Hinds PW, Levine AJ. The p53 proto-oncogene can act as a suppressor of transformation. Cell 1989; 57: 1083-93

63   Olsen JC, Johnson LG, Wong-Sun ML, Moore KL, Swanstrom R, Boucher RC. Retrovirus-mediated gene transfer to cystic fibrosis airway epithelial cells: effect of selectable marker sequences on long-term expression. Nucl Acids Res 1993; 21: 663-9

64   Burns JC, Friedmann T, Driever W, Burrascano M, Yee J-K. Vesicular stomatitis virus G glycoprotein pseudotyped retroviral vectors: Concentration to very high titer and efficient gene transfer into mammalian and nonmammalian cells. Proc Natl Acad USA 1993; 90: 8033-7

Subject Index